Easy *Keto*

FOR DUMMIES

Simple & Affordable 5-Ingredient Recipes for Busy
People and Low Carb Lovers On a Budget

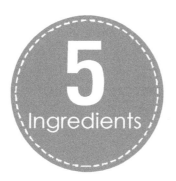

5
Ingredients

NANCY TRAVIS

Copyright ©2020 By Nancy Travis

TABLE OF CONTENT

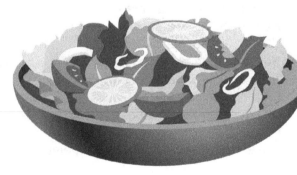

Introduction

Better cooking is a pathway to a better life. When we cook healthy and filling meals that are good for us, we teach ourselves valuable skills and improve our overall health. If we want to get healthy, we need to start by taking a good look at what we eat.

Tasty food isn't always good for us, but food that is good for us can be tasty. This is a lesson I learned at a very young age from my family, who have always been big believers in the idea that eating healthy doesn't have to mean bland, boring food. Learning this lesson made me all the more receptive to the ketogenic, or keto, diet. Rather than counting calories and confining ourselves to an endless parade of salads, keto lets us eat many of our favorite flavorful foods while still staying in shape.

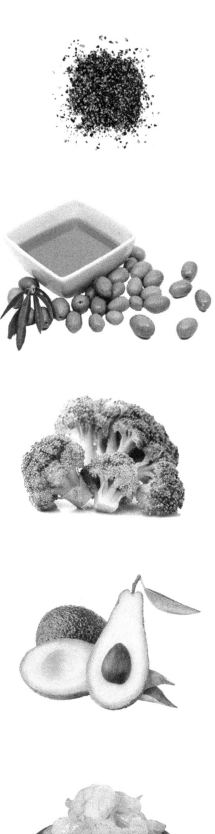

In this cookbook, I want to help you see that healthy meals don't have to be a chore to make or eat. You can achieve your weight loss goals or maintain your current level of fitness, and it doesn't have to take years of training or spending hours slaving away at the stove. You can make most of these meals in under 30 minutes! The five-ingredient recipes in this cookbook are as easy as they are delicious, full of easy-to-find and whole ingredients. There are recipes suitable for all kinds of diets, including vegetarian, vegan, dairy-free, and gluten-free, and they're perfect for chefs of any skill level.

We don't have to spend a lot of time in the kitchen or become professional chefs just to make healthy meals. In fact, it's possible to make tons of keto offerings with as few as five ingredients or less. This makes recipes quick and easy, allowing us to stick to our diets. Far from being another fad diet with lackluster results, the keto diet really works, and you'll be eating meals that would sound appealing even if you weren't on a diet at all.

If you're unfamiliar with the diet, you might be wondering what makes keto work? Can there really be a diet where you achieve weight loss by eating fat?

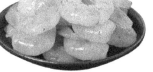

The Keto Diet Basics

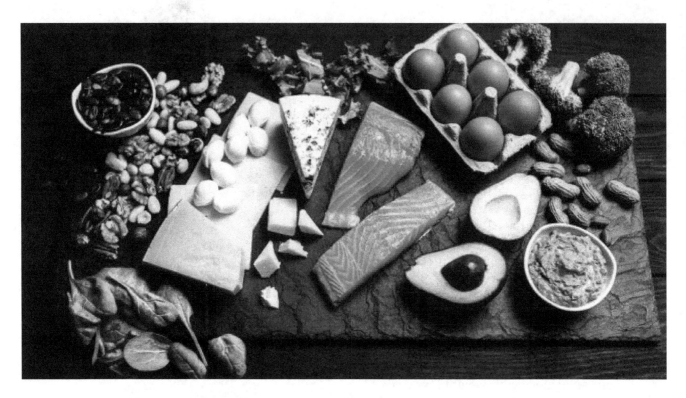

The keto diet is structured around the idea that excessive carbs cause us to gain weight. When we reduce the number of carbs in our diet through mindful eating habits, we enter a state of ketosis. In ketosis, our bodies switch over to using excess fat as an energy source, which leads to rapid weight loss. In this state, we will also find ourselves more energized than we were when we relied on carbs for our fuel.

Because we are eliminating a primary source of calories from our diet, we need to replace it with another type of food. On keto, this is accomplished by eating a higher number of fats. Far from being bad for us like we've always been told, fats can actually help us lose weight. Studies show that eating a high amount of healthy fats in our diets "helps slow down the rate at which your stomach empties during digestion" (Frank, 2016, para. 6), keeping us feeling fuller for longer. Fats give us the energy we need to keep ourselves going on a low-carb diet without tiring out or consuming too few calories to stay healthy.

Advantages of Keto

Keto's incorporation of fats into the diet means that it's rare to feel quite as hungry as you might on a calorie-restricting diet. The body digests fat slower than it breaks down carbs. This means that as long as you are eating enough fat, you will get consistent, long-lasting energy rather than the sharp peaks and dips of a high-carb diet. In addition, keto allows you to eat a lot of foods that would otherwise be banned in a traditional diet. There are still some restrictions about the kinds of fats you can have, but the keto diet is generally regarded as one of the tastier diets.

Another advantage of keto is that there's no need to write down the calories of every single meal and try to budget them. Keto doesn't require you to measure calorie counts at all. Instead, you only have to pay attention to your macronutrients, or macros, and the only hard limit is restricting your carb intake.

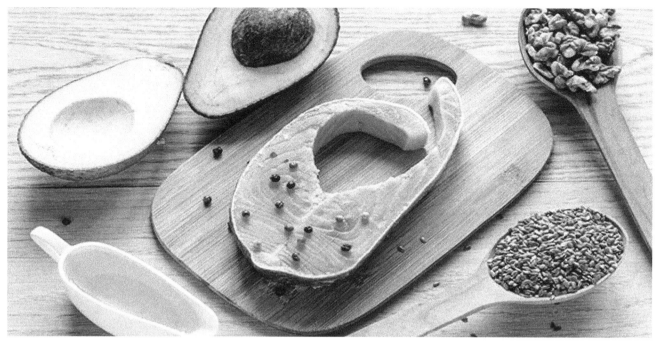

Ketosis and the Keto Flu

The one major disadvantage that could steer people away from the keto diet is the keto flu. This often involves light fatigue, headaches, dizziness, and other flu-like symptoms that are commonly reported at the beginning of the diet but which fade away over time. When you first enter ketosis, it is possible that you will feel some of these symptoms. However, if you are careful about how quickly you jump into a keto diet, you can drastically reduce the symptoms of the keto flu and avoid this period entirely.

Eating plenty of salt and drinking lots of water can really cut down on the likelihood of "catching" the keto flu. This keeps more water in your body, which reduces the risk of dehydration and can help push back against headaches and dizziness. Make sure to get plenty of fat in your diet on the first few days. Easing yourself into the diet can help you avoid these symptoms as well, so it's okay to eat a few medium-carb foods so long as you work them out of your diet later on.

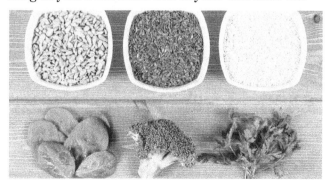

Macros of Keto Diet

Having a successful keto diet is all about hitting the right macros. For the best chances at success, you should track your carb, fat, and protein intake.

Keeping an eye on your carbs is the most important rule of keto. On a standard keto diet, you generally want to aim for no more than 15-20 grams of net carbs per day, and no more than 10 percent of your diet should be carbs. Eating along these guidelines should help you reach a state of ketosis and start burning fat. It's important to note that net carbs are a little different than the total carb count. They can be found by taking the total carbs and subtracting any fiber and sugar alcohols that are in the food, as your body does not digest these the same way it does normal carbs.

It's also important to make sure you're eating enough fats. The typical recommendation is around 70-80% of your diet should be made of fats, but more than that is fine. If you feel hungry at any point, you may need to increase the number of fats in your diet.

A moderate amount of protein is good for the keto diet. It should make up about 20% of your diet. Eating too much protein can interfere with your body's ability to use fats for fuel, so don't go overboard on steak and chicken.

For help tracking your macros and other important measurements on a keto diet, use our keto planner journal.

3

Food items	Date:_____ Week:_____ Keto Phrase:_____ Your Goal:_____					
	Mon					
	Breakfast	Lunch	Dinner	Snack	Trotal	Fasting time
Recipes						
Fat						
Protein						
Carbs						
Calories						
Liquid						
Exercise						
Ketosis reading						
Weight						
How you feel						
Self assessment						

Types of Fats

On keto, the types of fats you eat are just as important as the amount. There are "healthy fats" and "unhealthy fats," and you want to make sure the vast majority of your fats come from healthy sources. High amounts of monounsaturated and polyunsaturated fats like Omega-3s are great for you, while saturated fats and especially trans fats should be kept to a minimum. If you are having trouble reaching your fat macros, you can use an MCT oil supplement, which is common on the keto diet.

Monounsaturated fats are healthier than their counterparts. These oils generally remain liquid at room temperature and can be stored in the pantry. Monounsaturated fats include olive oil, avocado oil, and the fats from nuts. Polyunsaturated fats are generally safe too, and you can get them primarily from fish like salmon and tuna. Saturated fats come from animals and are commonly found in fatty cuts of meat and dairy products. Trans fats should be almost entirely avoided. These are man-made fats most commonly found in unhealthy snacks like cookies and chips.

Increasing the amount of healthy oils you use and consume is a great way to get good fats into your diet. Oil is great for sautéing food, and it's a common ingredient in most keto dressings and sauce recipes.

Tips for Keto Success

Succeeding on keto is easy as long as you stick to a high-fat, low-carb diet, but there are still some ways you can improve your experience. Some dieters find it useful to use ketone test strips, which will tell you when you're in ketosis. Others add a healthy amount of exercise into the mix, which becomes a lot easier with the energy keto gives you.

If your weight loss plateaus at any point before you've reached a healthy weight, you might not be eating enough fat. Try increasing the amount in your meals or adding MCT oil supplements to your diet.

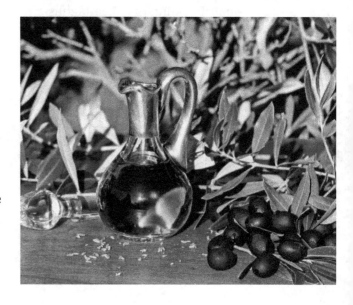

What to Eat on Keto Diet?

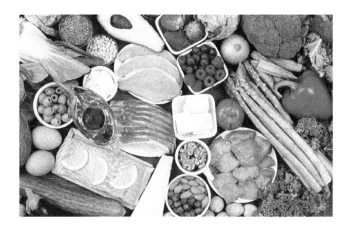

Eating on a keto diet is fairly easy, as the types of foods you want to eat and the ones you need to stay away from are mostly obvious. If you're eating a high-fat and low-carb diet, you want to eat plenty of fatty foods like fish, oil, nuts, cheese, avocado, and similar items. You also want to avoid the carb-heavy foods like bread, pasta, and rice, including sugary foods like soda, candy, and cake.

The process is complicated a bit by hidden sugars, which you might be eating without even knowing. On keto, naturally occurring sugars can kick you out of ketosis just the same as added sugars can. While you might think of fruits as healthy options, they can actually contain a lot of sugar, as can many dressings, sauces, and low-fat dairy products. In order to avoid accidental slip-ups, here's a quick guide you can use to identify the foods you can safely eat and the ones you should pass over.

Foods to Enjoy

Just about all natural meat and seafood can be safely incorporated into a keto diet. They are both very low in carbs, often containing no net carbs at all, so you can eat them with little worry of going over your carb limit. The only thing to potentially watch out for is the amount of saturated fat you're consuming. Seafood is high in healthy fats, but red meat tends to have more saturated fat in it. So just keep an eye on how often you have it. Protein should also be kept to a moderate amount on keto, so while it's fine to have meat or seafood for one or two meals each day, you should also include plenty of fat in the rest of your diet.

Some dairy is okay on keto as well. The main concern is the amount of sugar in dairy, either naturally occurring or as added sugars. Typically, dairy products made with whole milk have less sugar. Most cheeses are fine, as are low- or no-sugar varieties of yogurt, cream cheese, heavy cream, and sour cream.

Most nuts and seeds are fine for a keto diet as well. Pecans, Brazil nuts, and macadamia nuts are especially low in net carbs. Having a handful of nuts and seeds is a great keto-friendly snack so long as you can keep it to just a handful. Even small amounts of carbs can add up if you eat too many.

It's important to keep a close eye on your fruit consumption on a keto diet. Many fruits are high in sugar, but you can still have a little bit of fruit if you're smart about what you choose. Fruits like limes, lemons, tomatoes, and most berries like raspberries and strawberries are fine in moderation. Avocados are often a staple of the keto diet. On top of their low sugar content, they also have plenty of fat.

Vegetables are generally lower in sugar and therefore safer, though there are a few exceptions. Some great keto-friendly vegetables include lettuce, spinach, kale, cauliflower, broccoli, bell peppers, mushrooms, zucchini, celery, and eggplant.

No matter what you eat, consider the quality of your food. Look for grass-fed and free-range products, and spring for organic ingredients whenever possible. You should also try to incorporate fermented foods into your diet, as they support good gut health and good digestion.

Here's a quick breakdown of different types of foods that fit right into a keto diet, along with their macros per 100 grams.

Protein:
- Chicken: 23 g protein, 12 g fat, 0 g carbs
- Beef: 26 g protein, 19 g fat, 0 g carbs
- Pork: 26 g protein, 14 g fat, 0 g carbs
- Eggs: 13 g protein, 10 g fat, <1 g carbs
- Tuna: 30 g protein, 1 g fat, 0 g carbs
- Salmon: 25 g protein, 14 g fat, 0 g carbs
- Shrimp: 22 g protein, 2 g fat, 2 g carbs
- Crab: 17 g protein, 1 g fat, 0 g carbs

Fruits and vegetables:
- Strawberries: <1 g protein, <1 g fat, 6 g carbs
- Raspberries: 1 g protein, <1 g fat, 10 g carbs
- Blackberries: 1 g protein, <1 g fat, 9 g carbs
- Lemons: 1 g protein, <1 g fat, 7 g carbs
- Limes: <1 g protein, <1 g fat, 7 carbs
- Avocados: 2 g protein, 15 g fat, 8 g carbs

Fats:
- Olive oil: 0 g protein, 98 g fat, 0 g carbs
- Coconut oil: 0 g protein, 91 g fat, 0 g carbs
- Avocado oil: 0 g protein, 98 g fat, 0 g carbs
- Ghee: <1 g protein, 97 g fat, 0 g carbs

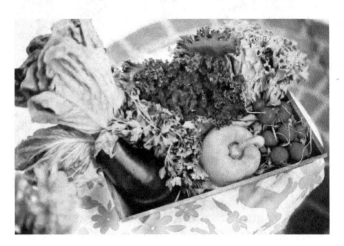

Foods to Avoid

Most natural meat and seafood options are safe, but watch out for additives and marinades. These can add unwanted sugars to the meal. Stay away from anything breaded or covered in a sugary sauce, and watch out for cured meats like ham and prosciutto, as sugar is usually involved in the curing process.

You want to avoid having too many dairy products in your diet, as even whole milk contains some naturally occurring sugars. Steer clear of low-fat dairy products especially, as these often have added sugar, and always remember to check the label before buying. Instead of regular milk, swap dairy out for unsweetened coconut milk or almond milk for a similar taste without all of the sugar.

While nuts and seeds are usually a safe choice if they are eaten in moderation, there are a few that are higher in carbs, like pistachios and

cashews. Also, watch out for those that come with added seasonings like honey-roasted peanuts or nuts that are mixed in with other foods, like trail mix. These varieties can add extra sugar. So long as you stick to plain or lightly salted varieties, you should be in the clear.

The vast majority of fruits are either heavily restricted or completely disallowed on a keto diet. Any fruit with high sugar is a bad idea. This includes apples, bananas, grapes, watermelon, mango, and pineapple, to list some of the biggest offenders. Vegetables are mostly safe, but there are some notable exceptions. Try to avoid eating starchy vegetables like potatoes, sweet potatoes, and corn. Parsnips and carrots aren't great either, and onions should be used sparingly.

Here are some foods to leave off of your keto meal plans and their carb macros per 100 grams.

Starches and grains:
- Pasta: 30 g carbs
- Cereal: 84 g carbs
- Rice: 32 g carbs
- Oats: 67 g carbs
- Quinoa: 65 g carbs
- Flour: 76 g carbs
- Bread: 56 g carbs
- Potatoes: 20 g carbs
- Corn: 22 g carbs

Sugary foods and drinks:
- Soda and other fountain drinks: 14 g carbs
- Fruit juice: 13 g carbs
- Low-fat milk: 8 g carbs
- Chocolate milk: 13 g carbs
- Cake: 42 g carbs
- Pastries: 35 g carbs
- Candy: 89 g carbs

Legumes:
- Beans: 24 g carbs
- Peas: 14 g carbs
- Lentils: 16 g carbs

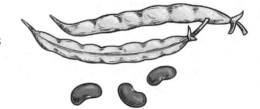

Processed, unhealthy fats and oils:

- Vegetable oil
- Sunflower oil
- Safflower oil
- Canola oil
- Soybean oil
- Grapeseed oil
- Corn oil
- Shortening
- Margarine
- Any hydrogenated or partially hydrogenated oils

Fruits:

- Bananas: 27 g carbs
- Grapes: 18 g carbs
- Dates: 74 g carbs
- Mangos: 16 g carbs
- Apples: 12 g carbs
- Watermelon: 10 g carbs
- Pineapple: 11 g carbs
- Raisins: 68 g carbs

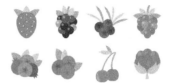

Keto Pantry Essentials

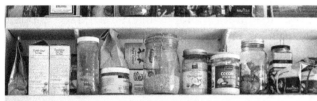

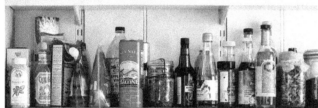

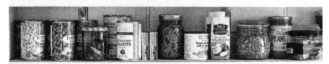

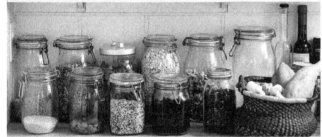

Keeping your fridge and pantry keto-friendly is just as important as keeping your meals keto-friendly. It's a good idea to make sure you have many common ingredients on hand. It's also a smart choice to rid your pantry of foods that aren't compliant with the keto diet. This helps reduce temptations and ensures that when you go to make a meal or grab a snack, you're only grabbing keto-friendly ingredients.

Clear Out All the High-Carb Items

Keeping high-sugar foods around is a recipe for disaster. The more temptations you have in your house, easily accessible, the harder it will be to stick to the keto diet. A pantry and fridge full of high-carb foods only undermines your efforts to stick to healthy eating.

Go through your pantry and remove anything with an excessive amount of carbs. This could be anything from rice, to boxes of pasta, to cans of beans, to chips and other snacks. When you've rounded up all of these items, try to get rid of them in a way that doesn't waste food. Donate the non-perishables to a local shelter or food bank, or give them to friends and other members of your community. Even though you can't eat it, this food can still help people who need it. Doing something good with this food can make it easier to part with.

Cooking Staples

While there are many ingredients that are keto-friendly, there are some you will find popping up over and over again in different recipes. These keto staples are great to have at the ready. You can safely add them to each week's grocery list so you know you always have access to them. Here are some foods you might want to keep around.

Meal Ingredients	Snacks	Oils and Supplements
No sugar added broth	Low-card nuts	Olive oil
Coconut flour	Canned tuna	Vegetable oil
Almond flour	Pork rinds	Avocado oil
Stevia or swerve sweetener	Olives	Ghee
Mayonnaise	Cheese crisps	Mct oil
Unsweetened cacao powder	Almond butter	Cooking spray

Kitchen Equipment

Alongside reworking your fridge and pantry, you might need to do some work on the equipment half of your kitchen. It pays off to be prepared, and part of prep work is making sure you have the right tools for the job. Without the right equipment, you're going to have trouble cooking all the recipes that make keto such a great and versatile diet.

Must-Have Equipment

A food scale is mandatory for properly following recipes. Food scales give you precision in your measurements. They also help you portion your food so you don't end up making much more or much less than you anticipated.

A good cast iron pan will get you far in the kitchen. It is a reliable tool you'll use for all manner of frying, sautéing, and even baking, so it's a worthwhile purchase.

Some appliances are great to have around in general but are especially useful for keto. A spiral slicer can turn all manner of vegetables into thin pasta-like spirals. This is often used to turn low-carb veggies like zucchini into a pasta replacement. Food processors will save you plenty of time, as you can quickly dice and combine ingredients. An electric hand mixer is a great purchase as well. It's invaluable for baking, and it's got plenty of cooking uses as well.

Don't let your knives fall behind either. You want to have a good set of reliable knives for chopping up ingredients without difficulty. You also want to keep these knives sharp, so investing in a knife sharpening stone is a good idea too.

Finally, a multi-cooker is a must-have addition to your cooking equipment. It lets you bake, grill, roast, steam, fry, deep fry, boil, and simmer, all with a single appliance. This is an incredibly helpful tool in the kitchen that will be the star of countless dinners.

Additional Equipment

There are a few more items that might be nice to have around the kitchen, though they're not exactly necessities. Silicone baking mats are super versatile non-stick cooking sheets that are perfect for everything from low-carb pizza to making a batch of cheese crisps. Silicone muffin trays are just as useful for making sugar-free baked goods.

It's also a good idea to keep some solid food storage options around. Make sure you have reliable, sturdy storage containers for leftovers. Mason jars are also good for storing dressings and sauces.

Safety Tips

If you're a little inexperienced with cooking, it's important to know proper knife safety. Keep your knives sharp to improve their efficiency and to reduce the risk of them slipping while cutting. Make sure to cut on a stable surface, and try to keep the ingredient you're cutting flat against the cutting board so it doesn't slide out of your hand. Always cut or peel away from yourself, never towards, and go slow to avoid any injuries. You should also make sure to store your knives so that the blades aren't sticking out. A knife block works best.

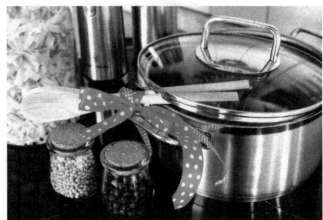

5-Ingredient Keto Easy and Quick Cooking Guide

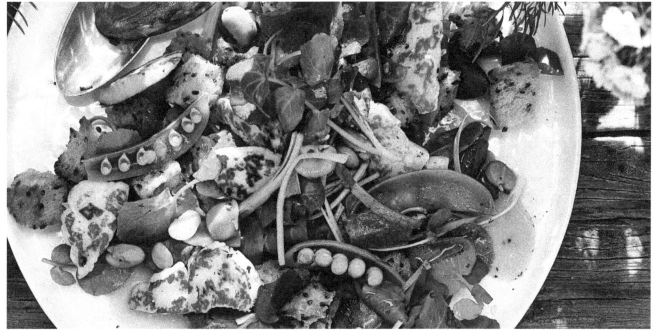

It almost sounds too good to be true, but it's possible to make tons of meals with just five ingredients. Keeping the ingredients list brief ensures that no recipe gets too complicated. It also helps ease the temptation of the "easy" high-carb meals that we're better off leaving behind. If cooking at home takes less time and is much better for you than grabbing fast food or heating up a ready-made meal full of sugars, there's much less temptation to eat something you shouldn't.

While these five-ingredient meals are already fairly easy to prepare and cook, there are some steps you can take to make the process even easier.

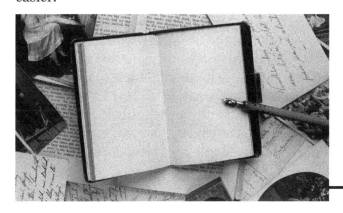

Meal Planning

Meal planning can be the difference between sticking to a keto diet and caving to temptation because you simply have no idea what to do for dinner tonight. When you plan your meals in advance, you can ensure you're getting enough variety in your diet, and you're more likely to cook meals that genuinely excite you. It's very simple to make a meal plan. You only need to choose a few meals you'd like to cook during the week, accounting for leftovers. Make sure to account for your daily macro goals when deciding on each day's meal plan.

Now that you know what you want to make this week, you can write out your grocery list. This keeps you from forgetting any crucial ingredients at the store. It also means you can get away with going to the store just once or twice each week, which can save a lot of time. When you do have to go, your trips are made more efficient by being able to follow your list. Don't forget to pick up a few of the basic keto staples while you're there!

Five Ingredient Cooking Tricks

Cooking meals with just five ingredients comes with quite a few benefits. The first and most obvious is that mealtime becomes a simpler affair. Recipes are shorter and easier to complete, so whether you are getting home from a long day of work or enjoying a lazy weekend, you can make amazing meals without spending hours in the kitchen. Planning your meals ahead of time can make the process even speedier, as can doing some light prep work in advance. This might mean grilling chicken at the start of the week so you have it ready for use in other meals, or it could mean putting together whole meals on the weekends and just heating up leftovers throughout the week. Cooking in bulk on the weekends and refrigerating or freezing the leftovers is a great way to get some prep work done.

Narrowing the number of ingredients can help you save money, especially when there's overlap between the recipes you choose to make. If you make three chicken recipes, you can go to the store and buy the big pack of chicken breasts, which costs significantly less than buying a pack of chicken, a pack of beef, and a pack of pork. It's still a good idea to have some variety, but when you can, cook recipes with similar ingredients to help you avoid unnecessary spending. You might even be able to save the leftover bits and pieces from one recipe and use them in another. For example, excess cut up bell peppers from a morning omelet could go into an afternoon salad. This reduces food waste and speeds up prep work.

If you know you won't have much time to cook, there's nothing wrong with buying frozen ingredients. Frozen food can be stored for a long time and only needs to be defrosted before use, which means you can keep ingredients around for a while until you need them.

Feel free to get creative with seasoning as well. If you're getting a bit bored of a recipe, adding in some spices can completely change the flavor. This can take a meal from a tired staple to a new, exciting favorite.

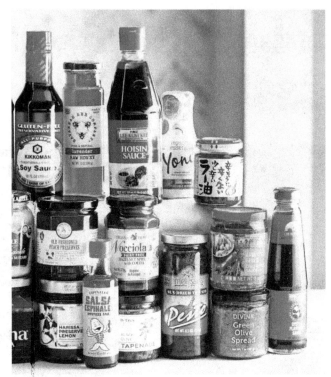

Pointers for the Cooking Process

When you're cooking, it's incredibly important that you read the recipe through before starting any meal. You want to get a good idea of all of the instructions before you start. This gives you a good idea of your next steps and helps you practice good time management.

It can also help to take out all of your ingredients right at the beginning of a recipe. This keeps you from rooting around in the fridge while something starts burning on the stove. It also reduces the risk of leaving an ingredient out because you forgot about it.

While no one likes the clean-up process, it's better to get it done sooner rather than later. Clean as you cook, and you'll save yourself a lot of work after dinner. Put ingredients you've already used away while your food is in the oven, and wipe down cutting boards and counters after use. This has the added benefit of reducing the risk of touching surfaces contaminated with raw meat or other potentially harmful ingredients. Luckily, these five-ingredient recipes are fairly light on clean-up, so you shouldn't have too much trouble.

Tips and Tricks

Whether you're a newbie in the kitchen or you're an old pro looking to change your dieting habits, it doesn't hurt to brush up on your skills. Here are some tips and tricks you can use to your advantage.

Storage Tips

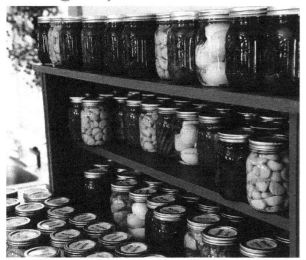

If you choose to cook meals in bulk, make sure you're storing your food properly. Choose air-tight containers and make sure you're eating leftovers before they have a chance to go bad. Freeze meals if you don't think you'll use them in a few days so you can keep them around longer.

Last-Minute Substitutions

No matter how well prepared you try to be, it's inevitable that at some point you're going to realize you completely ran out of an ingredient or you forgot to pick it up at the store. When you're looking for a substitution, make sure that your new ingredient is just as keto-friendly as the original recipe's choice.

It's not possible to list every single food substitution, but here are a few keto friendly ones that might help next time you're in a pinch. If you're out of butter, avocado makes for a creamy substitute. Mayo can be swapped out for Greek yogurt in most recipes. You can use lemon juice in place of vinegar. If you're missing a spice, check and see what you have in your pantry. A little salt, pepper, and garlic powder is a great seasoning combination for many meals.

Leftovers

Don't underestimate how useful it is to have leftovers around. Double up a recipe to get a few extra meals out of it for half the work. You can even repurpose leftovers into a completely different meal—for example, leftover chicken might become part of a casserole or the meat in your zoodles Bolognese. Get creative and keep your leftovers from becoming too repetitive.

How to Use a Five Ingredient Cookbook

As you look through the following recipes, you'll get a sense for just how easy cooking healthy meals can be. Since they all have just five or fewer recipes, there shouldn't be anything too intimidating no matter your current skill level. These recipes will help you eat healthy every day and get a jumpstart on finding success with the keto diet.

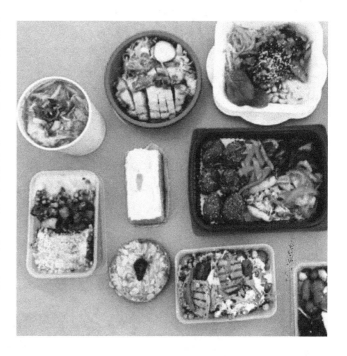

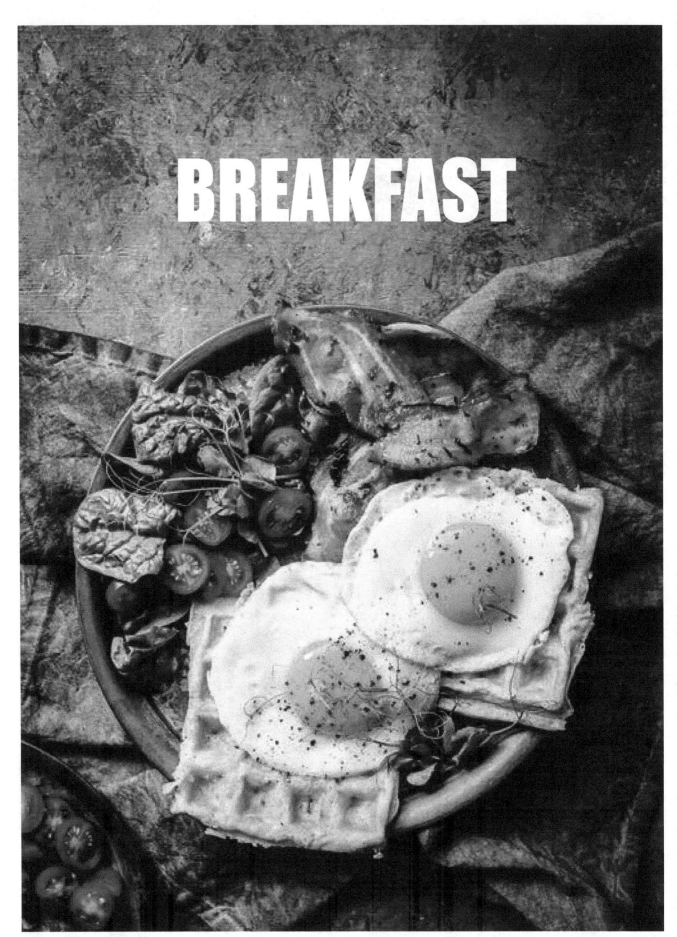

BREAKFAST

BREAKFAST EGG MUFFINS

Macros: Fat 63% | Protein 32% | Carbs 5%

Prep time: 10 minutes | Cook time: 25 minutes | Serves 6

1. Preheat the oven to 400°F (205°C).
2. Add the bacon strips in a skillet over medium heat and cook for about 5 minutes until crispy.
3. Transfer to a plate lined with paper towels and set aside. Reserve the bacon grease in the skillet.
4. In a bowl, stir together the beaten eggs and spinach. Set aside.
5. Grease 6 muffin tin cups with reserved bacon grease, then line each cup with a strip of bacon.
6. Spoon the egg mixture to the muffin cups evenly and top with Cheddar cheese. Season with salt and pepper.
7. Bake in the preheated oven for 15 minutes until completely set.
8. Remove from the oven and cool for 5 minutes before serving.

TIP: You can store the leftovers in a sealed airtight container in the fridge for up to 4 days.

PER SERVING
calories: 101 | fat: 7.1g | protein: 8.2g | net carbs: 1.1g

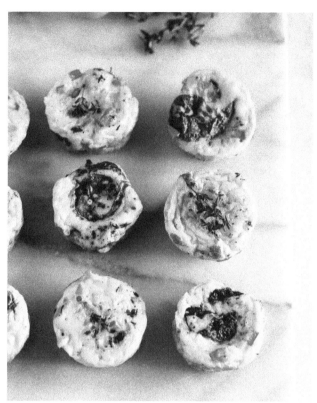

Ingredients:

6 large eggs, beaten

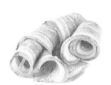

6 bacon strips

¼ cup Cheddar cheese, shredded

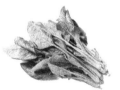

Handful of fresh spinach, chopped

FROM THE CUPBOARD:

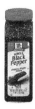

Sea salt and black pepper, to taste

SPECIAL EQUIPMENT:

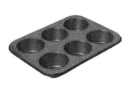

A 6-cup muffin tin

SAVORY HAM AND CHEESE WAFFLES

Macros: Fat 71% | Protein 28% | Carbs 1%

Prep time: 10 minutes | Cook time: 10 minutes | Serves 2

1. Preheat the waffle iron and set aside.
2. Crack the eggs and keep the egg yolks and egg whites in two separate bowls.
3. Add the butter, baking powder, basil, and salt to the egg yolks. Whisk well. Fold in the chopped ham and stir until well combined. Set aside.
4. Lightly season the egg whites with salt and beat until it forms stiff peaks.
5. Pour the egg whites into the bowl of egg yolk mixture. Allow to sit for about 5 minutes.
6. Lightly coat the waffle iron with the olive oil. Slowly pour half of the mixture in the waffle iron and cook for about 4 minutes. Repeat with the remaining egg mixture.
7. Remove from the waffle iron and serve warm on two serving plates.

TIP: To make this a complete meal, serve it with a cup of unsweetened almond milk.

PER SERVING
calories: 636 | fat: 50.2g | protein: 45.1g | net carbs: 1.1g

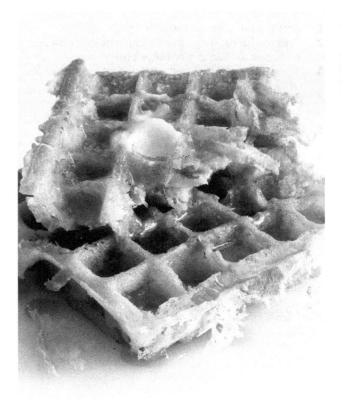

Ingredients:

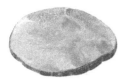

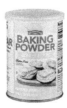

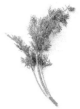

| 2 ounces (57 g) ham steak, chopped | 2 ounces (57 g) Cheddar cheese, grated | 8 eggs | 1 teaspoon baking powder | Basil, to taste |

FROM THE CUPBOARD:

SPECIAL EQUIPMENT:

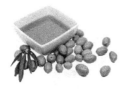

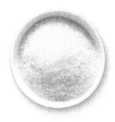

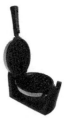

| 12 tablespoons butter, melted | Olive oil, as needed | 1 teaspoon sea salt | A waffle iron |

SHRIMP AND ARUGULA SALAD

Macros: Fat 84% | Protein 9% | Carbs 7%

Prep time: 10 minutes | Cook time: 0 minutes | Serves 8

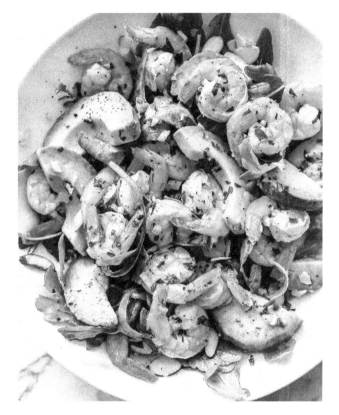

1. Make the dressing: In a bowl, stir together the olive oil, lemon juice, sea salt, and pepper.
2. Mix the avocado, shrimp, and arugula in a separate bowl. Pour over the dressing and stir to combine.
3. Divide the salad among eight serving plates and garnish with lemon wedges.

TIP: Mixing in the chopped cilantro can give this salad a unique twist.

PER SERVING
calories: 258 | fat: 24.2g | protein: 6.1g | net carbs: 4.1g

Ingredients:

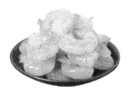

2 pounds (907 g) shrimp, cooked and peeled

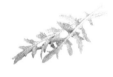

16 cups arugula, chopped

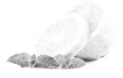

4 lemons, 2 juiced and 2 cut to serve

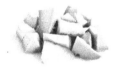

2 avocados, diced

FROM THE CUPBOARD:

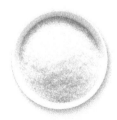

Sea salt and black pepper, to taste

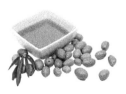

8 tablespoons olive oil

EASY BACON AND ARTICHOKE OMELET

Macros: Fat 81% | Protein 16% | Carbs 3%

Prep time: 10 minutes | Cook time: 10 minutes | Serves 4

1. Add the heavy cream, beaten eggs, and bacon in a bowl, whisking until combined fully. Set aside.
2. Heat the olive oil in a large skillet over medium-high heat. Fry the onion for about 3 minutes until tender.
3. Slowly pour the egg mixture into the skillet, tilting it to spread evenly. Cook for 2 minutes, then using a rubber spatula to lift the edges allowing uncooked portion to flow underneath. Top with the artichoke hearts and flip the omelet over. Cook for an additional 3 to 4 minutes, or until the omelet is almost set. Flip it again to make sure the artichoke heats are on top.
4. Transfer the omelet to a plate and slice into quarters. Sprinkle with salt and pepper before serving.

TIP: You can store the omelet in a sealed airtight container in the fridge for up to 3 days. It is not recommended to freeze.

PER SERVING
calories: 434 | fat: 39.3g | protein: 17.1g | net carbs: 3.1g | fiber: 2g

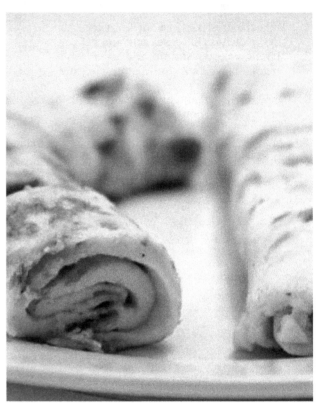

Ingredients:

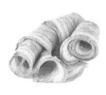

8 bacon slices, cooked and chopped

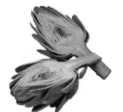

½ cup chopped artichoke hearts, canned and packed in water

6 eggs, beaten

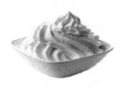

2 tablespoons heavy whipping cream

¼ cup onion, chopped

FROM THE CUPBOARD:

Sea salt, to taste

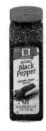

Freshly ground black pepper, to taste

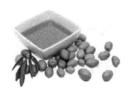

1 tablespoon olive oil

CLASSIC SPANAKOPITA FRITTATA

Macros: Fat 80% | Protein 17% | Carbs 3%

Prep time: 10 minutes | Cook time: 3 to 4 hours | Serves 8

1. Grease the bottom of the slow cooker insert with the olive oil lightly.
2. Stir together the beaten eggs, feta cheese, heavy cream, spinach, and garlic until well combined.
3. Slowly pour the mixture into the slow cooker. Cook covered on LOW for 3 to 4 hours, or until a knife inserted in the center comes out clean.
4. 4.Remove from the slow cooker and cool for about 3 minutes before slicing.

TIP: Blanching the spinach can give it a desired and uniform texture.

PER SERVING
calories: 254 | fat: 22.3g | protein: 11.1g | net carbs: 2.1g | fiber: 0g | cholesterol: 364mg

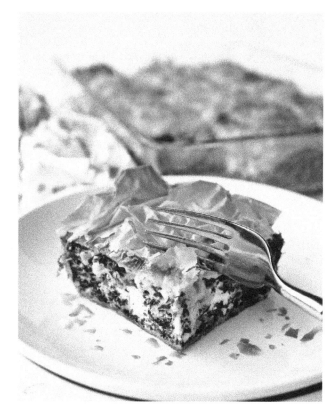

Ingredients:

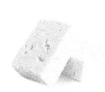

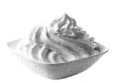

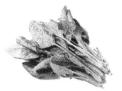

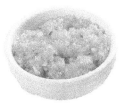

| 12 eggs, beaten | ½ cup feta cheese | 1 cup heavy whipping cream | 2 cups spinach, chopped | 2 teaspoons garlic, minced |

FROM THE CUPBOARD:

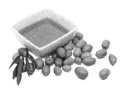

1 tablespoon extra-virgin olive oil

SAUSAGE STUFFED BELL PEPPERS

Macros: Fat 71% | Protein 22% | Carbs 7%

Prep time: 15 minutes | Cook time: 4 to 5 hours | Serves 4

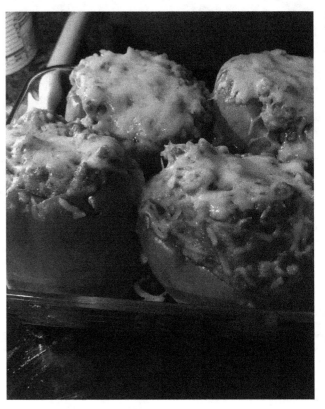

1. Add the coconut milk, eggs, and black pepper in a medium bowl, whisking until smooth. Set aside.
2. Line your slow cooker insert with aluminum foil. Grease the aluminum foil with 1 tablespoon olive oil.
3. Evenly stuff four bell peppers with the crumbled sausage, and spoon the egg mixture into the peppers.
4. Arrange the stuffed peppers in the slow cooker. Sprinkle the cheese on top.
5. Cook covered on LOW for 4 to 5 hours, or until the peppers are browned and the eggs are completely set.
6. Divide among four serving plates and serve warm.

TIP: Chicken, turkey, or ground beef can be used for the filling.

PER SERVING
calories: 459 | fat: 36.3g | protein: 25.2g | net carbs: 7.9g |fiber: 3g | cholesterol: 376mg

Ingredients:

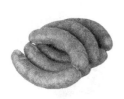

1 cup breakfast sausage, crumbled

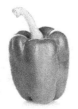

4 bell peppers, tops cut off and seeds removed

½ cup coconut milk

6 eggs

1 cup cheddar cheese, shredded

FROM THE CUPBOARD:

½ teaspoon freshly ground black pepper

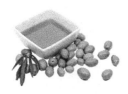

1 tablespoon extra-virgin olive oil

SLOW COOKER ASPARAGUS WITH DILL

Macros: Fat 72% | Protein 25% | Carbs 3%

Prep time: 10 minutes | Cook time: 3 to 4 hours | Serves 8

1. Grease the bottom of the slow cooker insert with the olive oil lightly.
2. Stir together the beaten eggs, coconut milk, dill, salt, and pepper in a medium bowl. Fold in the bacon and asparagus, then blend well.
3. Slowly pour the mixture into the greased slow cooker. Cook covered on LOW for about 3 to 4 hours.
4. Remove from the slow cooker and serve on a platter.

TIP: Blanching the asparagus can give it a smoother texture and an irresistible flavor.

PER SERVING
calories: 228 | fat: 18.3g | protein: 14.1g | net carbs: 1.9g |fiber: 1g | cholesterol: 281g

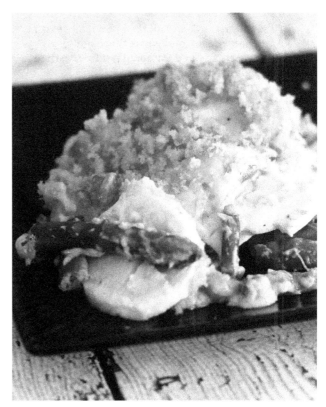

Ingredients:

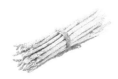

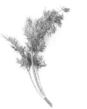

| 2 cups asparagus spears, chopped | 10 eggs, beaten | ¾ cup coconut milk | 2 teaspoons fresh dill, chopped | 1 cup cooked bacon, chopped |

FROM THE CUPBOARD:

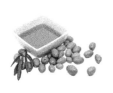
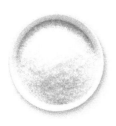
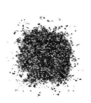

| 1 tablespoon extra-virgin olive oil | ½ teaspoon salt | ¼ teaspoon freshly ground black pepper |

CHIA BLUEBERRY PUDDING

Macros: Fat 75% | Protein 16% | Carbs 9%

Prep time: 15 minutes | Cook time: 0 minutes | Serves 2

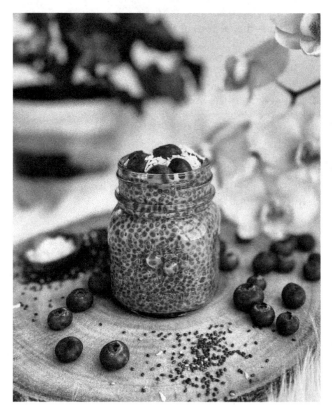

1. In a medium bowl, add all the ingredients except for the blueberries, and whisk thoroughly.
2. Let the mixture stand for about 5 minutes, then whisk again.
3. Wrap the bowl in plastic and refrigerate for at least 1 hour, preferably overnight.
4. Remove from the refrigerator and let stand at room temperature for a few minutes. Stir the pudding one more time and then scatter the blueberries on top before serving.

TIP: Any keto fruit, like strawberries or raspberries, can be substituted for the blueberries in this recipe.

PER SERVING
calories: 244 | fat: 20g | protein: 9.8g | net carbs: 6g | fiber: 21.9g | sugar: 1.8g

Ingredients:

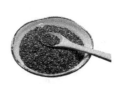

12 tablespoons chia seeds

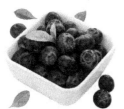

¼ cup blueberries

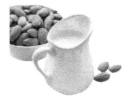

3 cups unsweetened almond milk

FROM THE CUPBOARD:

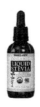

4 to 6 drops stevia

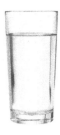

1 cup water

BLUEBERRY ALMOND FLAXSEED PUDDING

Macros: Fat 78% | Protein 15% | Carbs 7%

Prep time: 20 minutes | Cook time: 0 minutes | Serves 4

METHOD:
1. In a medium heatproof bowl, add the almonds and flaxseeds.
2. Put the water in a pot and bring it to a boil. Pour the hot water into the bowl with almonds and flaxseeds.
3. Add the lemon juice, and glucomannan powder, then stir to incorporate.
4. Pulse the almond mixture in a food processor until smooth. Transfer the mixture to an airtight container, and add the blueberries. Mix well and set aside to cool for about 5 minutes.
5. Once cooled, stir the mixture one more time and seal the container. Place in the fridge for 5 hours, preferably overnight.
6. Remove the pudding from the fridge. Let stand at room temperature for a few minutes, and serve.

TIP: You can top the pudding with any low-carb fruit, such as strawberries or raspberries.

PER SERVING
calories: 229 | fat: 20g | protein: 8.6g | net carbs: 3.7g | fiber: 10.6g | sugar: 2.1g

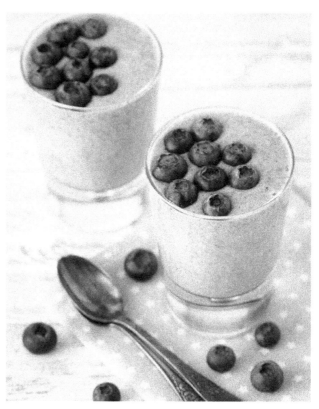

Ingredients:

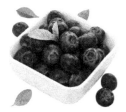

¼ cup frozen blueberries

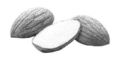

1 cup unsalted raw almonds

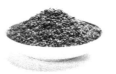

½ cup flaxseeds

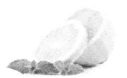

2 tablespoons lemon juice

2 teaspoons glucomannan powder

FROM THE CUPBOARD:

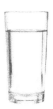

3 cups water

PUMPKIN MUFFINS WITH ALMOND MILK

Macros: Fat 84% | Protein 11% | Carbs 5%

Prep time: 10 minutes | Cook time: 30 minutes | Serves 12

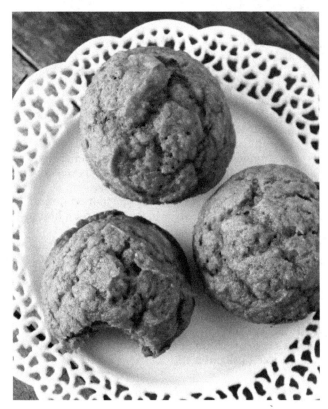

1. Preheat the oven to 350°F (180°C). Line a muffin pan with 12 paper liners and set aside.
2. Blend the coconut oil, stevia, pumpkin, almond milk, flaxseeds, almond flour, and vanilla extract in a blender until it forms a smooth batter.
3. Evenly divide the batter into the 12 paper liners. Arrange the muffin pan in the preheated oven and bake until a toothpick inserted in the center comes out clean, for about 30 minutes.
4. Remove from the oven and cool for 8 minutes before serving.

TIP: The canned pumpkin puree can be used as a substitute for pumpkin in this recipe.

PER SERVING
calories: 120 | fat: 11.2g | protein: 3.2g | net carbs: 1.7g | fiber: 1.9g | sugar: 0g

Ingredients:

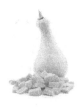

½ cup pumpkin, pitted and diced

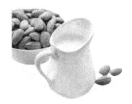

½ cup unsweetened almond milk

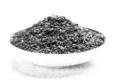

¼ cup ground flaxseeds

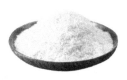

1 cup almond flour

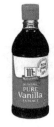

½ teaspoon vanilla extract

FROM THE CUPBOARD:

¼ cup coconut oil

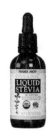

¼ teaspoon stevia

SPECIAL EQUIPMENT:

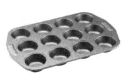

A 12-cup muffin pan

CHEESY CHICKEN AND AVOCADO OMELET

Macros: Fat 78% | Protein 20% | Carbs 2%

Prep time: 10 minutes | Cook time: 10 minutes | Serves 2

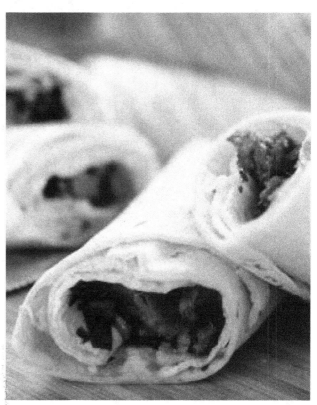

1. Beat the eggs and heavy cream in a medium bowl until smooth and creamy.
2. In a frying pan over medium heat, heat the olive oil. Add the egg mixture and cook for about 2 minutes, or until the eggs are just barely set. Using a rubber spatula to lift the edges allowing uncooked portion to flow underneath, then cook for about 4 minutes more.
3. Sprinkle the chicken and avocado on top. Season as needed with salt and pepper.
4. Cut the omelet in half, then transfer to two serving plates. Top with the cheese and serve.

TIP: To add a good dose of fat and flavor, serve it with the bacon and mayo.

PER SERVING
calories: 197 | fat: 17.3g | protein: 9.3g | net carbs: 1.1g | fiber: 2g

Ingredients:

4 large eggs

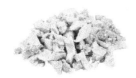

½ cup cooked chicken, chopped

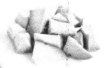

1 avocado, diced

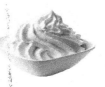

¼ cup heavy (whipping) cream

¼ cup crumbled feta cheese

FROM THE CUPBOARD:

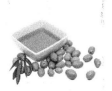

2 tablespoons extra-virgin olive oil

Sea salt, to taste

Freshly ground black pepper, to taste

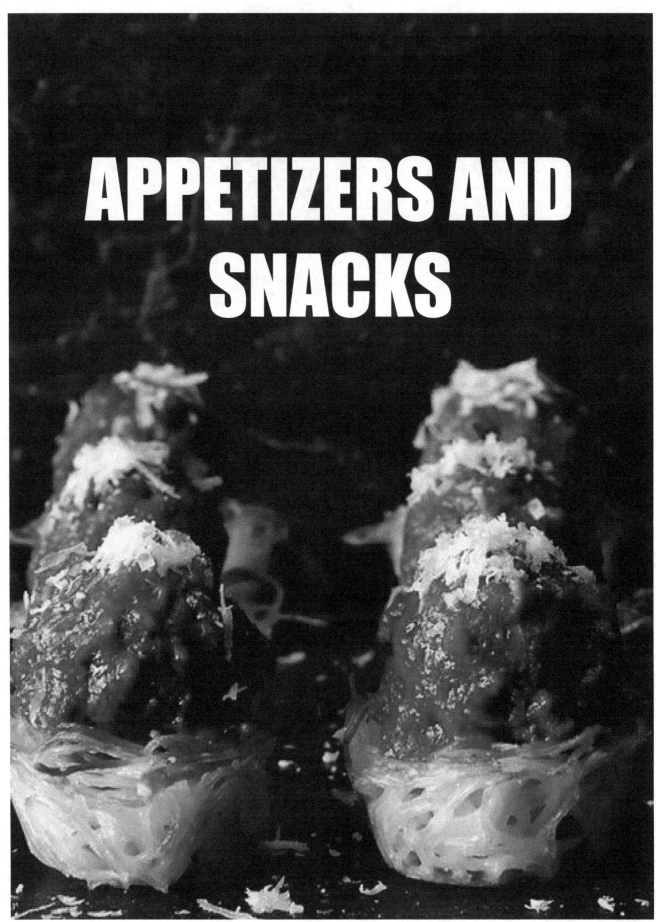

APPETIZERS AND SNACKS

WALNUT-CRUSTED GOAT CHEESE WITH THYME

Macros: Fat 82% | Protein 16% | Carbs 2%

Prep time: 10 minutes | Cook time: 0 minutes | Serves 4

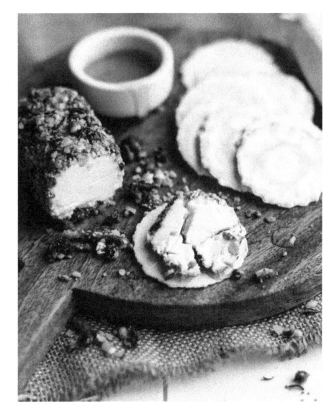

1. In a food processor, process the walnuts, thyme, parsley, oregano, and pepper until chopped thoroughly.
2. Transfer the walnut mixture to a plate and roll the goat cheese in the nut mixture, pressing so the cheese is coated completely.
3. Cover the cheese with plastic wrap and refrigerate for at least 1 hour.
4. Remove from the refrigerator and slice to serve.

TIP: The snack can be prepared a day ahead; the flavors only enhance with time.

PER SERVING
calories: 311 | fat: 28.2g | protein: 12.5g | net carbs: 1.9g

Ingredients:

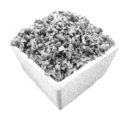

6 ounces (170 g) walnuts, chopped

8 ounces (227 g) goat cheese

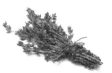

1 teaspoon fresh thyme, chopped

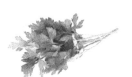

1 tablespoon parsley, chopped

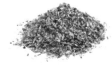

1 tablespoon oregano, chopped

FROM THE CUPBOARD:

¼ teaspoon black pepper

BACON-WRAPPED CHEESE STICKS

Macros: Fat 49% | Protein 47% | Carbs 4%

Prep time: 10 minutes | Cook time: 10 minutes | Serves 4

1. Heat 2 inches of olive oil for 3 to 4 minutes in a large skillet over medium-high heat.
2. Meanwhile, wrap one bacon strip around each piece of cheese, securing with a toothpick.
3. Using tongs, carefully put the bacon-wrapped cheese sticks in the skillet. Cook them for about 2 minutes per side until crispy, flipping occasionally.
4. Transfer to a plate lined with paper towels to drain off any excess grease. Cool for about 5 minutes before serving.

TIP: The temperature of olive oil should be about 350°F (180°C), preventing melting the Mozzarella cheese.

PER SERVING
calories: 275 | fat: 14.9g | protein: 32.2g | net carbs: 3.1g

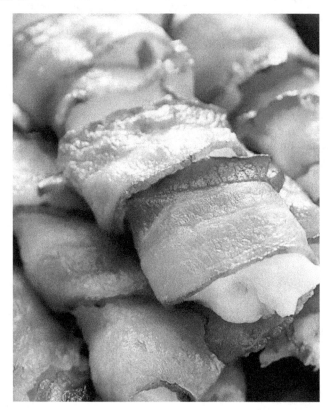

Ingredients:

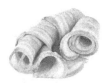

4 Mozzarella string cheese pieces, cut in half

8 bacon strips

FROM THE CUPBOARD:

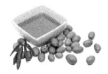

Olive oil, as needed

SPECIAL EQUIPMENT:

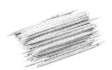

8 toothpicks, soaked for at least 30 minutes

SMOKED SALMON ROLL-UPS WITH ARUGULA

Macros: Fat 75% | Protein 21% | Carbs 4%

Prep time: 15 minutes | Cook time: 0 minutes | Serves 4

1. Combine the yogurt, cream cheese, and dill in a small bowl. Stir well until it is smooth.
2. Make the roll-ups: Divide evenly the mixture onto each salmon slice, spreading it all over. Arrange some arugula at one end of each salmon slice and roll up.
3. Divide the roll-ups among four serving plates. Drizzle a dash of olive oil on top for garnish and serve.

TIP: You can secure each roll-up with a toothpick to keep it from unrolling while cooking.

PER SERVING
calories: 244 | fat: 20.4g | protein: 13g | net carbs: 2.1g | fiber: 0g | sodium: 539mg

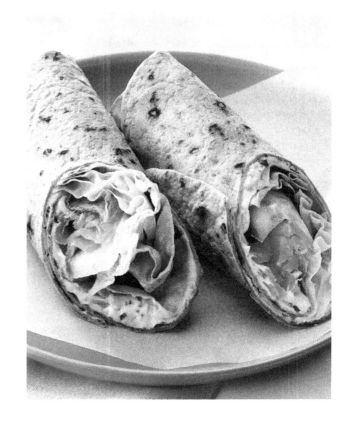

Ingredients:

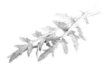

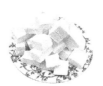

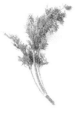

| 12 slices (½-pound / 227-g) smoked salmon | ¾ cup arugula | ¼ cup plain Greek yogurt | ½ cup cream cheese | 2 teaspoons fresh dill, chopped |

FROM THE CUPBOARD:

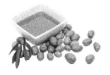

Olive oil, for garnish

GRILLED KALE LEAVES

Macros: Fat 87% | Protein 4% | Carbs 9%

Prep time: 10 minutes | Cook time: 5 minutes | Serves 4

1. Preheat the grill to medium-high heat and lightly grease the grill grates with the olive oil.
2. Make the dressing: Combine the garlic powder, lemon juice, and olive oil in a bowl, and whisk until the mixture is thickened.
3. Put the kale leaves in the bowl, and massage the dressing into the leaves with your hands. Lightly sprinkle with salt and pepper.
4. Grill the kale leaves on the preheated grill for about 2 minutes. Flip the leaves over and grill for 1 minute more until crispy.
5. Remove from the heat to a plate and serve hot.

TIP: You can use some spices and herbs of your choice for a unique taste other than the garlic powder.

PER SERVING
calories: 291 | fat: 28.3g | protein: 3.2g | net carbs: 5.9g | fiber: 3g | sodium: 38mg

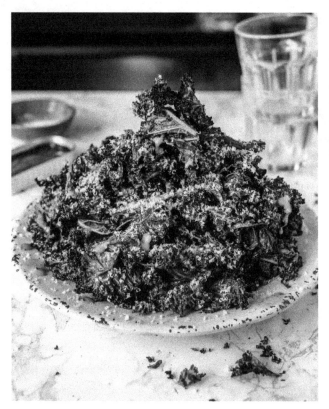

Ingredients:

½ teaspoon garlic powder

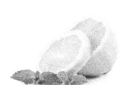

2 teaspoons freshly squeezed lemon juice

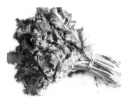

7 cups large kale leaves, thoroughly washed and patted dry

FROM THE CUPBOARD:

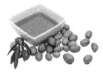

½ cup olive oil, plus more for greasing the grill grates

Sea salt, to taste

Freshly ground black pepper, to taste

CREAMED COCONUT SPINACH

Macros: Fat 86% | Protein 4% | Carbs 10%

Prep time: 10 minutes | Cook time: 20 minutes | Serves 4

1. Melt the butter in a frying pan over medium heat. Toss in the onions and fry for 2 minutes until translucent.
2. Add the coconut cream, vegetable broth, spinach, nutmeg, salt, and pepper. Cook for about 15 minutes, stirring occasionally, or until the sauce is thickened and the spinach is tender.
3. Transfer the creamed coconut spinach to serving bowls and serve warm.

TIP: The coconut oil can be substituted for the butter in this recipe.

PER SERVING
calories: 87 | fat: 8.3g | protein: 1g | net carbs: 2.1g | fiber: 1g | sodium: 60mg

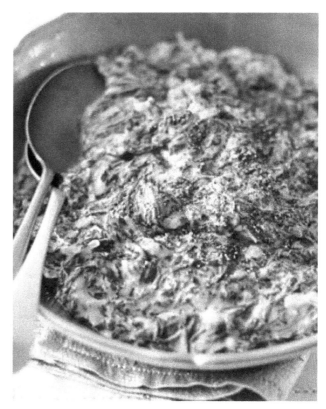

Ingredients:

¼ cup coconut cream

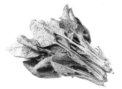
4 cups coarsely chopped spinach, thoroughly washed

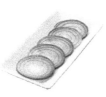
¼ onion, thinly sliced

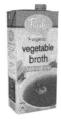
½ cup vegetable broth

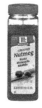
⅛ teaspoon ground nutmeg

FROM THE CUPBOARD:

1 tablespoon butter

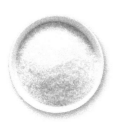
Pinch sea salt

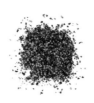
Pinch freshly ground black pepper

EASY GRILLED ASPARAGUS

Macros: Fat 75% | Protein 10% | Carbs 15%

Prep time: 5 minutes | Cook time: 5 minutes | Serves 4

1. Preheat the grill to high heat and lightly grease the grill grates with the olive oil.
2. Toss the asparagus in the olive oil in a medium bowl, then sprinkle with salt and pepper.
3. Grill the asparagus in the preheated grill for 2 to 4 minutes, flipping once, or to desired tenderness.
4. Remove from the heat and serve on plates.

TIP: To add more flavors to this meal, you can generously drizzle the melted butter on top of the grilled asparagus.

PER SERVING
calories: 83 | fat: 6.9g | protein: 2.2g | net carbs: 3g | fiber: 2g | sodium: 28mg

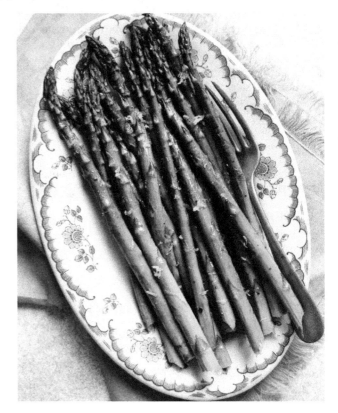

Ingredients:

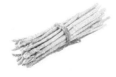

1 pound (454 g) fresh asparagus spears, woody ends snapped off

FROM THE CUPBOARD:

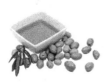

2 tablespoons olive oil, plus more for greasing the grill grates

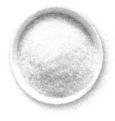

Sea salt, to taste

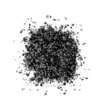

Freshly ground black pepper, to taste

CHEESY BACON FAT BOMBS

Macros: Fat 85% | Protein 15% | Carbs 0%

Prep time: 10 minutes | Cook time: 0 minutes | Makes 12 fat bombs

1. Line a baking sheet with parchment paper. Keep it aside.
2. Make the fat bombs: Combine the cream cheese, goat cheese, bacon, butter, and pepper in a medium bowl. Stir well to incorporate.
3. Scoop tablespoon-sized mounds of the mixture onto the baking sheet and roll into balls with your palm.
4. Transfer the fat bombs to the fridge for 1 hour until firm but not completely solid.
5. Remove from the fridge and let stand at room temperature for a few minutes before serving.

TIP: You can store the fat bombs in a sealed airtight container in the fridge for up to 2 weeks.

PER SERVING
calories: 87 | fat: 8.2g | protein: 3.4g | net carbs: 0g | fiber: 0g

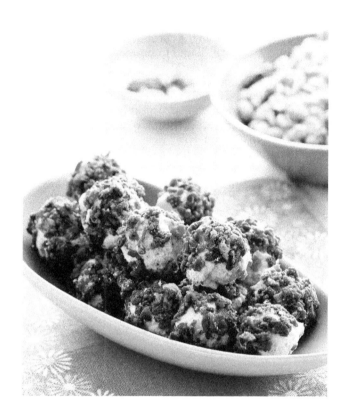

Ingredients:

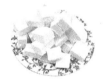

2 ounces (57 g) cream cheese, at room temperature

2 ounces (57 g) goat cheese, at room temperature

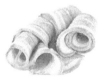

8 bacon slices, cooked and chopped

FROM THE CUPBOARD:

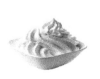

¼ cup butter, at room temperature

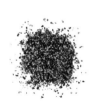

Pinch freshly ground black pepper

SIMPLE QUESO DIP

Macros: Fat 78% | Protein 18% | Carbs 4%

Prep time: 5 minutes | Cook time: 10 minutes | Serves 6

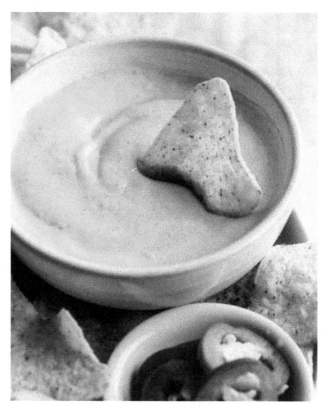

1. Add the garlic in a saucepan over medium heat, then slowly pour in the coconut milk and jalapeño pepper. Allow the liquid to simmer for about 3 minutes.
2. Add the goat cheese and keep whisking until the mixture is completely combined and smooth.
3. Add the Cheddar cheese, whisking continuously, or until the mixture is thickened and bubbling, about 1 to 2 minutes.
4. Remove from the heat to a serving bowl and serve warm.

TIP: To add more flavors to this dip, garnish it with a pinch more of cayenne.

PER SERVING
calories: 218 | fat: 18.9g | protein: 10g | net carbs: 2.1g | fiber: 0g

Ingredients:

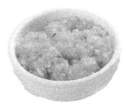

1 teaspoon garlic, minced

½ cup coconut milk

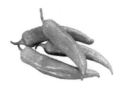

½ jalapeño pepper, seeded and diced

2 ounces (57 g) goat cheese, shredded

6 ounces (170 g) sharp Cheddar cheese, shredded

KETO ZUCCHINI HASH

Macros: Fat 77% | Protein 17% | Carbs 6%

Prep time: 10 minutes | Cook time: 20 minutes | Serves 1

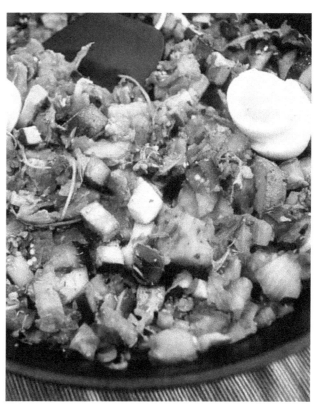

1. In a skillet over medium heat, add the bacon slices. Cook for about 5 minutes, flipping occasionally, or until desired crispness. Transfer to a bowl and set aside.
2. Heat the olive oil and sauté the onion for 3 minutes, stirring occasionally, or until the onion is translucent.
3. Toss in the zucchini and brown for 10 minutes until the zucchini is perfectly tender. Sprinkle the salt to season, then transfer to a platter and set aside.
4. Separate the egg into the skillet and cook for about 1 to 2 minutes until completely set, flipping once.
5. Spread the bacon slices and fried egg on top of the zucchini. Sprinkle the parsley on top for garnish and serve.

TIP: You can try any of your favourite veggies, such as cauliflower, kale, and Brussels sprouts.

PER SERVING
calories:415 | fat: 35.6g | protein: 17.4g | net carbs: 6.5g

Ingredients:

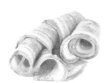

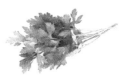

| 1 medium zucchini, diced | 2 bacon slices | ½ small onion, chopped | 1 egg | 1 tablespoon chopped parsley, for garnish |

FROM THE CUPBOARD:

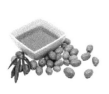

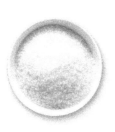

1 tablespoon olive oil   ¼ teaspoon salt

BACON CAPRESE SALAD

Macros: Fat 72% | Protein 26% | Carbs 2%

Prep time: 10 minutes | Cook time: 10 minutes | Serves 2

1. In a saucepan over medium heat, add the chopped bacon. Cook for about 5 minutes until crunchy, stirring occasionally.
2. Remove from the heat to a plate, and set aside.
3. Make the salad: Evenly place the tomato slices onto two serving platters. Top with the Mozzarella cheese slices and sprinkle with basil leaves, followed by the bacon slices.
4. Drizzle the olive oil and balsamic vinegar over the salad. Lightly season with sea salt before serving.

TIP: Store in a sealed airtight container in the fridge for 4 to 5 days.

PER SERVING
calories: 326 | fat: 26.3g | protein: 21g | net carbs: 1.4g

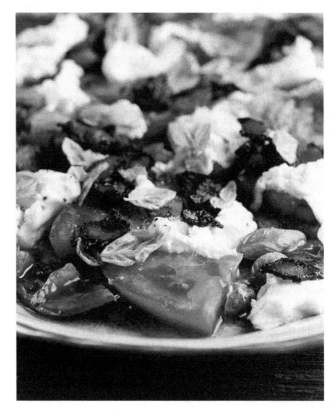

Ingredients:

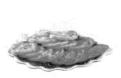

1 large tomato, sliced

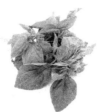

4 basil leaves

8 Mozzarella cheese slices

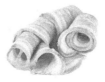

3 ounces (85 g) bacon, chopped

FROM THE CUPBOARD:

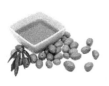

2 teaspoons olive oil

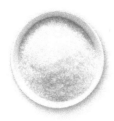

Sea salt, to taste

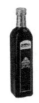

1 teaspoon balsamic vinegar

BROWNED SCALLOPS WITH LEMON BUTTER

Macros: Fat 84% | Protein 12% | Carbs 4%

Prep time: 5 minutes | Cook time: 10 minutes | Serves 4

1. In a bowl, combine the butter, garlic cloves, parsley, lemon juice, salt, and pepper. Stir well and set aside.
2. Preheat the oven to 450°F (235°C).
3. Heat the olive oil in a pan over medium heat until hot, then sear the scallops for about 30 seconds. Using tongs, flip the scallops and continue to cook for 30 seconds until lightly browned on both sides.
4. Remove from the heat to four serving plates. Top with a generous drizzle of butter mixture.
5. Bake in the preheated oven for about 5 minutes, or until the butter begins to bubble and foam.
6. Remove from the oven and serve warm.

TIP: Make sure to dry the scallops with paper towels before baking.

PER SERVING
calories: 271 | fat: 25.3g | protein: 7.9g | net carbs: 3.1g | fiber: 0g

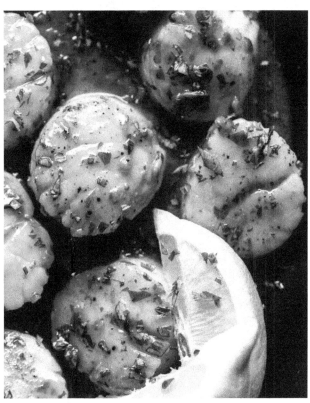

Ingredients:

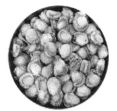

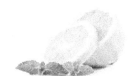

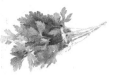

8 scallops   1 teaspoon lemon juice   2 garlic cloves   2 tablespoons fresh parsley, chopped

FROM THE CUPBOARD:

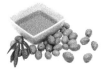

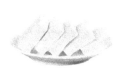

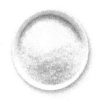

1 tablespoon olive oil   4¼ ounces (120 g) butter, at room temperature   1 teaspoon sea salt   ¼ teaspoon ground black pepper

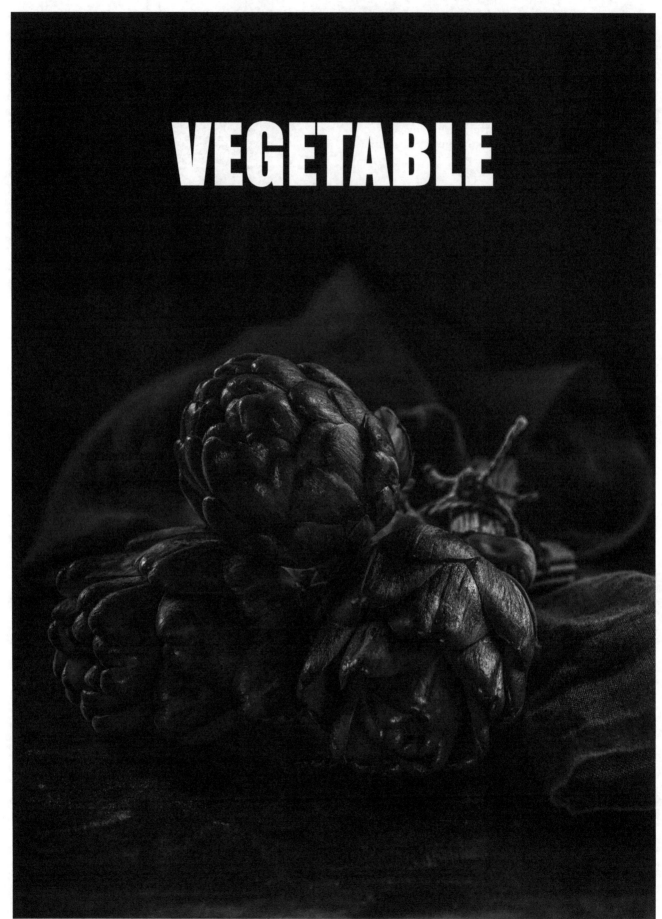

VEGETABLE

SPINACH AND FETA CHEESE FRITTATA

Macros: Fat 71% | Protein 23% | Carbs 6%

Prep time: 10 minutes | Cook time: 25 minutes | Serves 4

1. Preheat the oven to 350°F (180°C). Grease the bottom of a 2-quart casserole with olive oil and set aside.
2. Stir together the beaten eggs, salt, and pepper in a bowl until well combined. Fold in the feta cheese, spinach, and scallions. Mix well.
3. Slowly pour the egg mixture into the greased casserole, then sprinkle the halved cherry tomatoes on top.
4. Bake in the preheated oven for about 25 minutes until the top is golden brown.
5. Remove from the heat and let cool for 5 minutes before cutting into wedges.

TIP: To make this a complete meal, serve it with salad or steamed low-carb vegetables.

PER SERVING
calories: 447.3 | fat: 35.3g | protein: 26.3g | net carbs: 6.1g

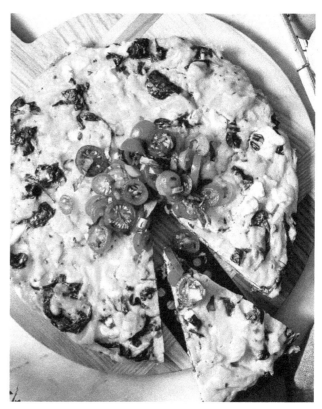

Ingredients:

10 eggs, beaten

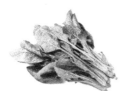

5 ounces (142 g) spinach, chopped

8 ounces (227 g) feta cheese, crumbled

4 scallions, diced

1 cup cherry tomatoes, halved

FROM THE CUPBOARD:

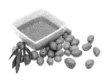

3 tablespoon olive oil

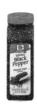

Salt and black pepper, to taste

CREAMY MUSHROOM SOUP

Macros: Fat 83% | Protein 9% | Carbs 8%

Prep time: 10 minutes | Cook time: 25 minutes | Serves 4

1. In a large saucepan over medium heat, add the butter and heat to melt.
2. Fold in the garlic cloves and sauté for 1 minutes until fragrant.
3. Stir in the mushrooms and sprinkle with salt and pepper. Cook for about 10 minutes.
4. Add the vegetable broth and bring to a rapid boil. Cover, and simmer gently on medium-low heat for 10 minutes.
5. Remove the pan from the heat and allow to cool slightly. Using an immersion blender to purée the soup until smooth.
6. Return the pan to the heat and add the crème fraiche. Cook for 2 minutes more until warmed through.
7. Divide the soup among four serving bowls and serve topped with the thyme leaves.

TIP: To add more flavors to this meal, serve it with a bowl of cauliflower rice.

PER SERVING
calories: 275 | fat: 25.3g | protein: 6.2g | net carbs:5.7 g

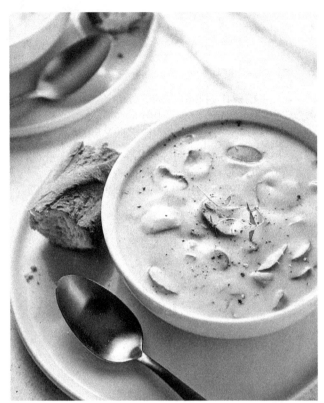

Ingredients:

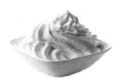

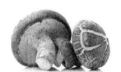

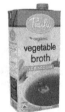

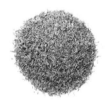

| 5 ounces (142 g) crème fraiche | 12 ounces (340 g) wild mushrooms, chopped | 2 garlic cloves, minced | 4 cups vegetable broth | 2 teaspoon thyme leaves |

FROM THE CUPBOARD: SPECIAL EQUIPMENT:

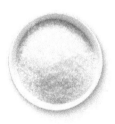

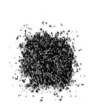

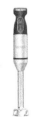

| ¼ cup butter | Salt and black pepper, to taste | An immersion blender |

STUFFED PORTOBELLO MUSHROOMS

Macros: Fat 77% | Protein 17% | Carbs 6%

Prep time: 10 minutes | Cook time: 20 minutes | Serves 2

1. Preheat the oven to 350°F (180°C). Line a baking sheet with parchment paper and set aside.
2. In a bowl, toss the lettuce in the olive oil. Set aside.
3. Using a spoon, stuff each mushroom cap with a considerable amount of the crumbled blue cheese.
4. Arrange the stuffed mushrooms on the baking sheet. Bake in the preheated oven for about 20 minutes, or until the cheese is melted.
5. Remove from the heat and allow to cool for 5 minutes. Serve the mushrooms with the lettuce on the side.

TIP: Any low-carb veggie can be used for the mushroom filling, and you can sprinkle the Mozzarella cheese on top.

PER SERVING
calories: 341 | fat: 29.3g | protein: 14.2g | net carbs: 5.3g

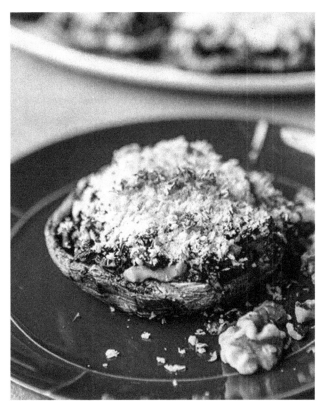

Ingredients:

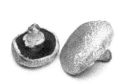

4 portobello mushrooms, stems removed

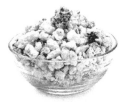

1 cup blue cheese, crumbled

2 cups lettuce

FROM THE CUPBOARD:

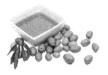

2 tablespoons olive oil

BROCCOLI AND CAULIFLOWER CASSEROLE

Macros: Fat 78% | Protein 17% | Carbs 5%

Prep time: 15 minutes | Cook time: 6 hours | Serves 6

1. Grease the bottom of the slow cooker insert with 1 tablespoon olive oil.
2. Put the cauliflower and broccoli into the slow cooker. Set aside.
3. Combine the coconut milk, almond flour, 1 cup of the gouda cheese, and pepper in a bowl, whisking until combined.
4. Pour the mixture over the cauliflower and broccoli, then sprinkle the remaining cheese on top.
5. Cook covered on LOW for about 6 hours until the vegetables are tender.
6. Let it cool for about 8 minutes, then serve.

TIP: The coconut flour can be substituted for the almond flour, just use 1 tablespoon coconut flour in the recipe.

PER SERVING
calories: 376 | fat: 32.3g | protein: 16.1g | net carbs: 6.1g | fiber: 6g | cholesterol: 32mg

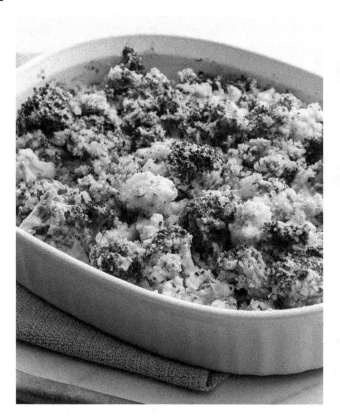

Ingredients:

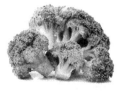

1 pound broccoli, cut into florets

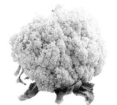

1 pound cauliflower, cut into florets

2 cups coconut milk

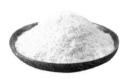

¼ cup almond flour

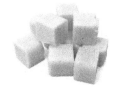

1½ cups shredded gouda cheese, divided

FROM THE CUPBOARD:

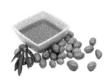

1 tablespoon extra-virgin olive oil

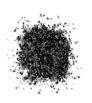

Pinch freshly ground black pepper

40 Vegetable

KALE WITH GARLIC AND BACON

Macros: Fat 67% | Protein 21% | Carbs 12%

Prep time: 15 minutes | Cook time: 6 hours | Serves 8

1. Coat the bottom of the slow cooker insert with 2 tablespoons bacon fat.
2. Put the bacon slices, kale, garlic, and vegetable broth into the slow cooker, then give the mixture a stir.
3. Cook covered on LOW for about 6 hours. When ready to serve, sprinkle the salt and pepper to taste.
4. Allow to cool for 5 minutes before serving.

TIP: Other keto vegetables, like bok choy or spinach, can be used as a substitute for kale.

PER SERVING
calories: 135 | fat: 10.3g | protein: 7.1g | net carbs: 4.1g |fiber: 3g | cholesterol: 17mg

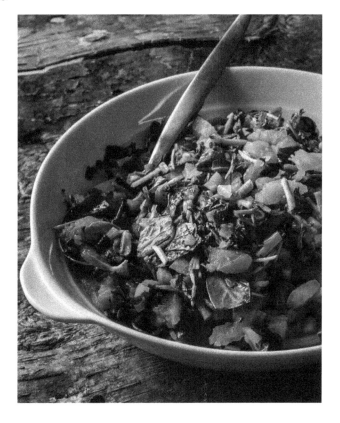

Ingredients:

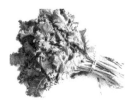

2 pounds (907 g) kale, rinsed and chopped roughly

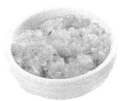

2 teaspoons garlic, minced

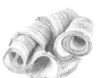

12 bacon slices, cooked and chopped

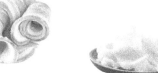

2 tablespoons bacon fat

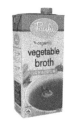

2 cups vegetable broth

FROM THE CUPBOARD:

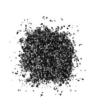

Salt and freshly ground black pepper, to taste

EASY SUMMER VEGETABLE MEDLEY

Macros: Fat 88% | Protein 3% | Carbs 9%

Prep time: 15 minutes | Cook time: 6 hours | Serves 6

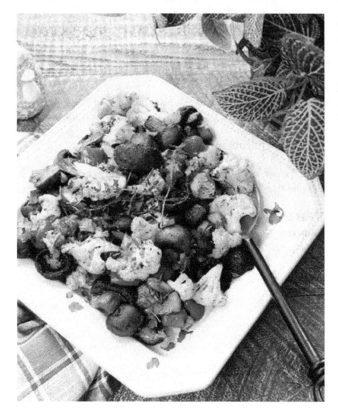

1. Stir together the olive oil, vinegar, salt, and thyme in a large bowl until well combined.
2. Fold in the zucchini, cauliflower, mushrooms, and bell pepper strips, then toss until the vegetables are coated thoroughly.
3. Put the vegetables into the slow cooker and cook covered on LOW for about 6 hours, or until the vegetables are tender.
4. Let stand for 5 minutes and serve warm on a plate.

TIP: The balsamic vinegar can be replaced with the low-carb vinegars, such as apple cider vinegar or red wine vinegar.

PER SERVING
calories: 186 | fat: 18.3g | protein: 1.2g | net carbs: 4.1g |fiber: 1g | cholesterol: 0mg

Ingredients:

2 zucchinis, diced into 1-inch pieces

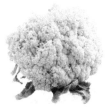

2 cups cauliflower florets

1 cup button mushrooms, halved

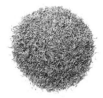

1 teaspoon dried thyme

1 yellow bell pepper, cut into strips

FROM THE CUPBOARD:

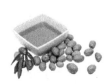

½ cup extra-virgin olive oil

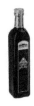

¼ cup balsamic vinegar

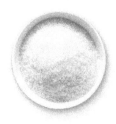

¼ teaspoon salt

ROASTED CAULIFLOWER AND AVOCADO HUMMUS

Macros: Fat 91% | Protein 4% | Carbs 5%

Prep time: 10 minutes | Cook time: 25 minutes | Serves 2

1. Preheat the oven to 450°F (235°C). Line a baking sheet with aluminum foil.
2. Arrange the cauliflower on the baking sheet, then drizzle 2 tablespoons olive oil over the cauliflower.
3. Place the baking sheet in the preheated oven and roast until the cauliflower is lightly browned, about 20 to 25 minutes.
4. Remove from the oven and set aside to cool for 5 minutes.
5. In a food processor, put the roasted cauliflower and remaining ingredients. Pulse until it reaches the desired hummus-like consistency.
6. Put the mixture into a bowl and cover with plastic wrap. Refrigerate for about 1 hour.
7. Remove from the refrigerator and allow to stand at room temperature for a few minutes. Season with salt and pepper, if desired.

TIP: To make this a complete meal, serve it with almond bread on the side.

PER SERVING
calories: 397 | fat: 40.6g | protein: 3.5g | net carbs: 4.3g

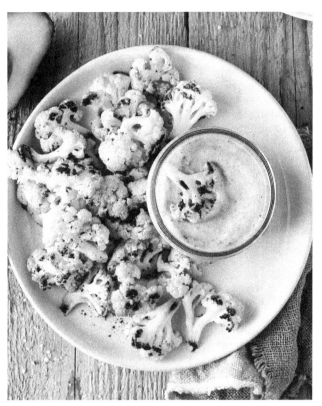

Ingredients:

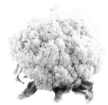

1 medium cauliflower, stem removed and chopped

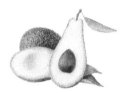

1 large Hass avocado, peeled, pitted, and chopped

2 garlic cloves

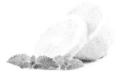

½ tablespoon lemon juice

FROM THE CUPBOARD:

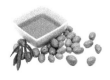

¼ cup extra virgin olive oil

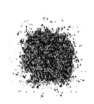

Sea salt and ground black pepper, to taste

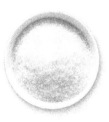

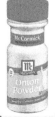

½ teaspoon onion powder

MARGHERITA MUSHROOM PIZZA

Macros: Fat 72% | Protein 20% | Carbs 8%

Prep time: 15 minutes | Cook time: 15 minutes | Serves 6

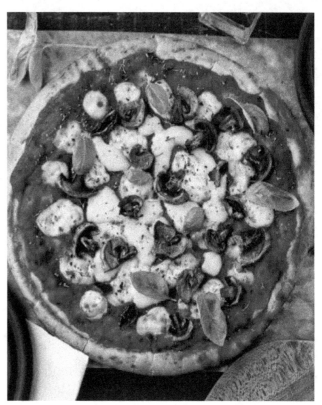

1. Preheat the oven to 350°F (180°C), and line a baking tray with aluminum foil. Set aside.
2. Combine the mushrooms, garlic, and olive oil in a medium bowl. Toss well until the mushrooms are fully coated.
3. Arrange the mushrooms (gill-side down) on the baking tray. Roast in the preheated oven for about 12 minutes, flipping once, or until the mushrooms are firm but tender.
4. Remove from the oven and pour the tomato sauce over the mushroom caps. Sprinkle the Mozzarella cheese on top.
5. Return the baking tray to the oven and roast for 1 to 2 minutes more, or until the cheese melts.
6. Remove from the oven and garnish with the chopped basil.

TIP: To add a good dose of fat and flavor, you can sprinkle the chopped Italian sausage or prosciutto on top of the mushrooms other than Mozzarella cheese.

PER SERVING
calories: 317 | fat: 25.3g | protein: 16.2g | net carbs: 6.1g | fiber: 3g

Ingredients:

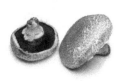

6 large portobello mushrooms, stems removed

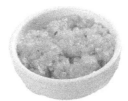

1 teaspoon garlic, minced

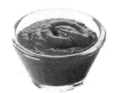

1 cup sugar-free tomato sauce

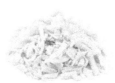

2 cups Mozzarella cheese, shredded

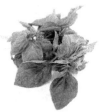

2 tablespoons chopped fresh basil, for garnish

FROM THE CUPBOARD:

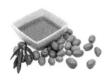

½ cup extra-virgin olive oil

CREAMY GREEN CABBAGE

Macros: Fat 87% | Protein 5% | Carbs 8%

Prep time: 5 minutes | Cook time: 12 minutes | Serves 4

1. In a skillet over medium-high heat, add the butter and heat to melt.
2. Toss in the sliced cabbage and fry for about 5 minutes until the edges start to brown, stirring occasionally.
3. Fold in the heavy whipping cream and mix well. Reduce the heat, cover, and allow to simmer for about 5 minutes more.
4. Season as needed with salt and pepper. Serve topped with the lemon zest and parsley.

TIP: The heavy whipping cream can be replaced with the unsweetened coconut milk, if you'd like to reduce your dairy intake.

PER SERVING
calories: 398 | fat: 38.3g | protein: 5.2g | net carbs: 8.1g | fiber: 5g

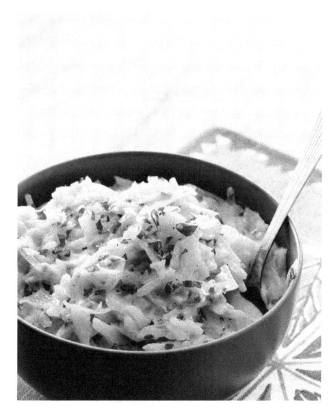

Ingredients:

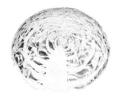

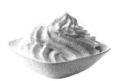

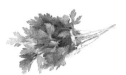

| 1½ pounds (680 g) green cabbage, thinly sliced | 1¼ cups heavy whipping cream | 1 tablespoon lemon zest | ½ cup fresh parsley, finely chopped |

FROM THE CUPBOARD:

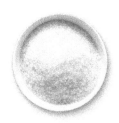

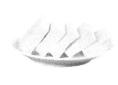

| Salt and pepper, to taste | 2 ounces (57 g) butter |

SEAFOOD AND FISH

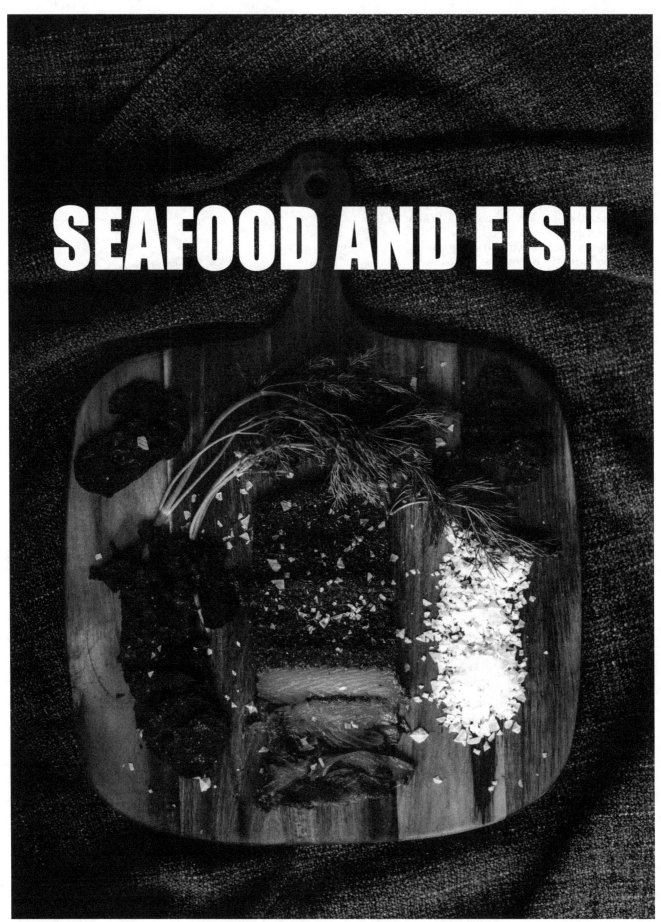

BAKED SOLE WITH ASIAGO CRUST

Macros: Fat 66% | Protein 28% | Carbs 6%

Prep time: 10 minutes | Cook time: 8 minutes | Serves 4

1. Preheat the oven to 350°F (180°C) and line a baking tray with parchment paper. Set aside.
2. In a small bowl, mix the cheese and ground almonds until well blended.
3. One at a time, drop the sole fillets in the whisked eggs, shaking off the excess, then coat in the almond mixture.
4. Arrange the sole fillets on the prepared baking tray, then rub each fillet with the coconut oil.
5. Place the baking tray in the preheated oven and bake for 8 minutes, or until the fish flakes easily with a fork.
6. Remove from the heat and serve on plates.

TIP: Store in an airtight container in the fridge for up to 4 days or in the freezer for up to one month.

PER SERVING
calories: 419 | fat: 31.3g | protein: 29.2g | net carbs: 3.1g |fiber: 3g

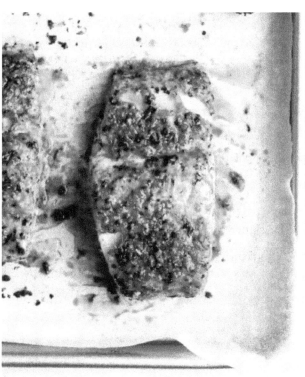

Ingredients:

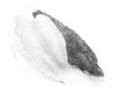

4 (4-ounce / 113-g) sole fillets, patted dry

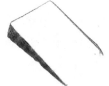

¼ cup Asiago cheese

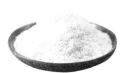

¾ cup ground almonds

2 eggs, whisked

FROM THE CUPBOARD:

2½ tablespoons coconut oil, melted

COCONUT HADDOCK WITH HAZELNUT

Macros: Fat 72% | Protein 26% | Carbs 2%

Prep time: 10 minutes | Cook time: 12 minutes | Serves 4

1. Preheat the oven to 400°F (205°C) and line a baking tray with parchment paper. Set aside.
2. In a bowl, rub the fillets with salt and pepper. Mix together the ground hazelnuts and coconut on a platter.
3. Dip the seasoned fillets in the nut mixture, pressing so the fillets are coated fully.
4. Arrange the fillets on the prepared baking tray and brush them with 2 tablespoons coconut oil.
5. Place the baking tray in the preheated oven and bake for about 12 minutes until flaky.
6. Transfer to four serving plates and serve warm.

TIP: You can substitute other nuts of your choice for the hazelnuts, such as almonds or walnuts.

PER SERVING
calories: 304 | fat: 24.3g | protein: 20.2g | net carbs: 1.1g | fiber: 3g

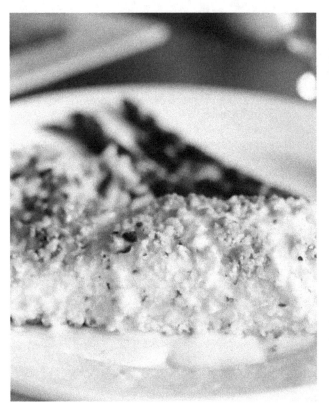

Ingredients:

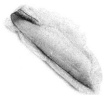

4 (5-ounce / 142-g) boneless haddock fillets, patted dry

¼ cup ground hazelnuts

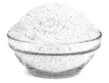

1 cup unsweetened coconut, shredded

FROM THE CUPBOARD:

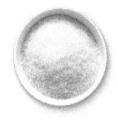

Sea salt and freshly ground black pepper, to taste

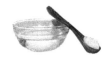

2 tablespoons coconut oil, melted

POACHED TROUT IN CREAM

Macros: Fat 75% | Protein 22% | Carbs 3%

Prep time: 10 minutes | Cook time: 20 minutes | Serves 4

1. Preheat the oven to 400°F (205°C).
2. In a bowl, season the fillets as needed with salt and pepper.
3. Arrange the seasoned fillets on a baking dish, and set aside.
4. Melt the butter in a saucepan over medium-high heat. Add the garlic and leek to fry for about 6 minutes until tender, stirring occasionally.
5. Pour the lemon juice and heavy cream into the saucepan, stirring continuously, and allow to boil until the sauce is thickened.
6. Pour the sauce over the fillets and transfer to the preheated oven. Bake for 10 to 12 minutes until the fish is flaky.
7. Remove from the oven and allow to cool for a few minutes before serving.

TIP: This meal can be eaten the way it is. However, you can serve it alongside the cauliflower rice.

PER SERVING
calories: 449 | fat: 37.3g | protein: 24.2g | net carbs: 4.1g | fiber: 1g

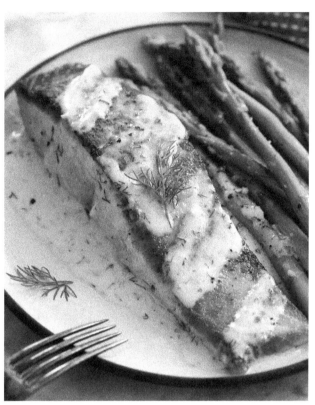

Ingredients:

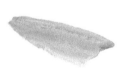
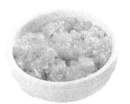
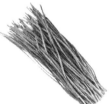
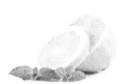
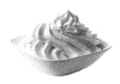

| 4 (4-ounce / 113-g) skinless trout fillets, patted dry | 1 teaspoon garlic, minced | 1 leek, thinly sliced and thoroughly washed | Juice of 1 lemon | 1 cup heavy whipping cream |

FROM THE CUPBOARD:

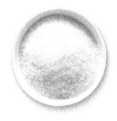
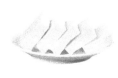

Sea salt and freshly ground black pepper, to taste   3 tablespoons butter

CREAMED SALMON WITH HERB

Macros: Fat 79% | Protein 19% | Carbs 2%

Prep time: 10 minutes | Cook time: 10 minutes | Serves 2

1. In a bowl, season the salmon fillets with ½ teaspoon of the tarragon and dill.
2. In a skillet over medium heat, heat the duck fat until it melts.
3. Stir in the salmon fillets and fry for 4 minutes per side until cooked through. Transfer to two serving plates and set aside.
4. Add the butter in the skillet and heat to melt. Stir in the remaining tarragon and dill, then cook for about 30 seconds. Fold in the heavy whipping cream and cook for 1 minute more, stirring occasionally, or until the sauce is warmed through.
5. Remove from the heat and evenly pour the sauce over the fillets, then serve.

TIP: This meal goes well with warm kale salad, cauliflower rice, or zucchini noodles.

PER SERVING
calories: 459 | fat: 40.4g | protein: 22.2g | net carbs: 1.51g

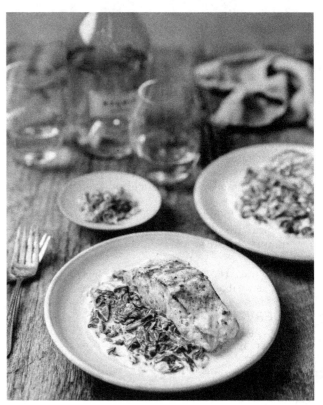

Ingredients:

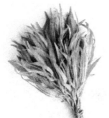
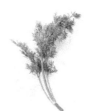
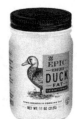
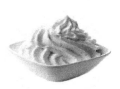

| 2 salmon fillets | 1 teaspoon tarragon, divided | 1 teaspoon dill, divided | 1 tablespoon duck fat | ¼ cup heavy whipping cream |

FROM THE CUPBOARD:

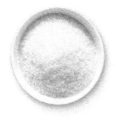
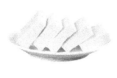

Sea salt and freshly ground black pepper, to taste   2 tablespoons butter

GRILLED SHRIMP WITH SAUCE

Macros: Fat 70% | Protein 24% | Carbs 6%

Prep time: 10 minutes | Cook time: 5 minutes | Serves 4

1. In a blender, add the ¼ cup olive oil, red onion, red wine vinegar, parsley, garlic cloves, salt and pepper. Process until the sauce is smooth, then set aside.
2. In a bowl, mix together the lime juice, 2 tablespoons olive oil, and shrimp. Place in the refrigerator to marinate for about 30 minutes.
3. Preheat the grill to medium heat and lightly grease the grill grates with the olive oil.
4. Transfer the marinated shrimp to the preheated grill. Cook for about 4 minutes, flipping occasionally.
5. Remove the shrimp from the grill to four serving plates. Pour the sauce over the shrimp and serve.

TIP: To make this a delicious meal, serve it with roasted asparagus with Parmesan.

PER SERVING
calories: 262 | fat: 20.4g | protein: 16.2g | net carbs: 3.6g

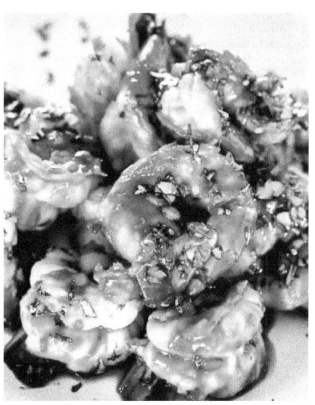

Ingredients:

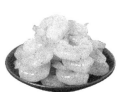
1 pound (454 g) shrimp, peeled and deveined

¼ cup red onion, chopped

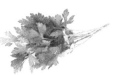
2 cups parsley

2 garlic cloves

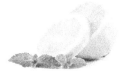
Juice of 1 lime

FROM THE CUPBOARD:

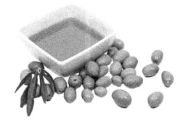
2 tablespoons olive oil, plus more for greasing the grill grates

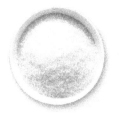
¼ cup olive oil

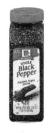
½ teaspoon salt

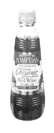
½ teaspoon pepper

¼ cup red wine vinegar

FUSS-FREE CRAB CAKES WITH LEMON JUICE

Macros: Fat 57% | Protein 25% | Carbs 18%

Prep time: 10 minutes | Cook time: 6 minutes | Serves 8

1. In a bowl, put all the ingredients except for the olive oil. Stir to incorporate.
2. Make the crab cakes: Scoop out 2 tablespoons of the meat mixture and shape into a patty with your palm, about ½ inch thick. Repeat with the remaining meat mixture. Set aside.
3. In a large frying pan over medium heat, heat the olive oil until sizzling. Add the crab cakes and fry gently for 3 minutes on each side until crisp and golden.
4. Transfer to a plate lined with paper towels. Let cool for 5 minutes before serving.

TIP: To add more flavors to this meal, you can also serve with the cocktail sauce on the side.

PER SERVING
calories: 84 | fat: 5.3g | protein: 5.4g | net carbs: 3.7g

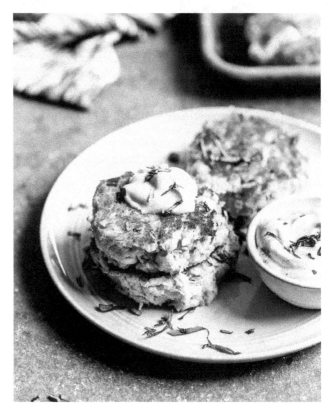

Ingredients:

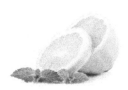

1 tablespoon lemon juice

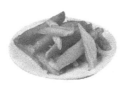

1 cup lump crab meat

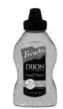

2 teaspoons Dijon mustard

1 egg, beaten

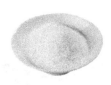

1½ tablespoons coconut flour

FROM THE CUPBOARD:

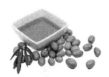

2 tablespoons olive oil

HAZELNUT CRUSTED SEA BASS

Macros: Fat 62% | Protein 35% | Carbs 3%

Prep time: 10 minutes | Cook time: 15 minutes | Serves 2

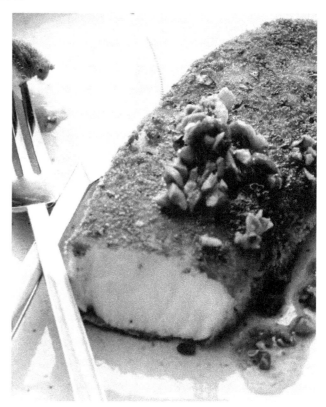

1. Preheat the oven to 425°F (220°C) and line a baking tray with parchment paper. Set aside.
2. In a bowl, rub the butter all over the fillets. Set aside.
3. Pulse the hazelnuts and cayenne pepper in a food processor until chopped thoroughly. Transfer the hazelnut mixture to a plate.
4. Dredge the fillets in the nut mixture so that both sides of each fillet are thickly coated.
5. Arrange the coated fillets on the baking tray. Bake in the preheated oven for 15 minutes, or until the fish flakes easily with a fork.
6. Remove from the oven and serve on plates.

TIP: To add more favors to this dish, you can sprinkle with a tasty tarragon and Parmesan cheese.

PER SERVING
calories: 453 | fat: 31.2g | protein: 40.2g | net carbs: 2.9g

Ingredients:

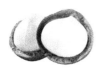

⅓ cup hazelnuts, roasted

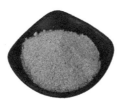

2 sea bass fillets

A pinch of cayenne pepper

FROM THE CUPBOARD:

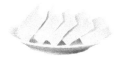

2 tablespoons butter, melted

SALMON WITH BROWNED BUTTER

Macros: Fat 75% | Protein 25% | Carbs 0%

Prep time: 10 minutes | Cook time: 20 minutes | Serves 4

1. Preheat the oven to 350°F (180°C). Line a baking tray with aluminum foil, then lightly coat the bottom of the baking tray with the olive oil.
2. In a bowl, rub the salmon fillets with salt and pepper, then transfer to the baking tray. Brush both sides of each fillet with 1 tablespoon olive oil.
3. Place the baking tray in the preheated oven and bake for 18 to 20 minutes until cooked through.
4. Meanwhile, heat the butter in a frying pan over medium heat, stirring occasionally, until the butter froths and brown flecks appear. Remove from the heat.
5. Remove the fillets from the oven to four serving plates. Pour the butter over the fillets evenly and sprinkle the thyme on top for garnish.

TIP: Do not overcook the butter in the frying pan, or it will turn dark.

PER SERVING
calories: 366 | fat: 30.3g | protein: 23.3g | net carbs: 0g | fiber: 0g

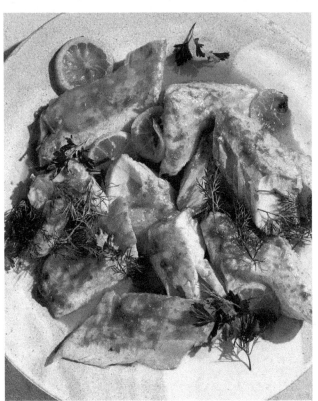

Ingredients:

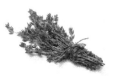

4 (4-ounce / 113-g) salmon fillets, patted dry

1 teaspoon chopped fresh thyme, for garnish

FROM THE CUPBOARD:

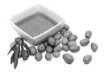

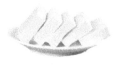

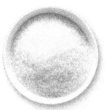

1 tablespoon extra-virgin olive oil, plus more for greasing the baking tray

⅓ cup butter

Sea salt and freshly ground black pepper, to taste

NUT CRUSTED HALIBUT

Macros: Fat 72% | Protein 27% | Carbs 1%

Prep time: 20 minutes | Cook time: 15 minutes | Serves 4

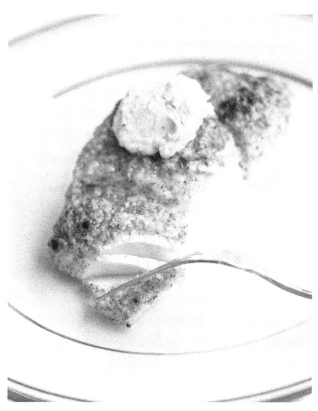

1. Preheat the oven to 400°F (205°C) and line a baking sheet with parchment paper. Set aside.
2. In a bowl, add the heavy whipping cream. In a separate bowl, mix the almonds and pecans together. Set aside.
3. On a clean work surface, lightly sprinkle the fillets with salt and pepper.
4. Dredge the seasoned fillets in the heavy cream and shake off the excess, then coat them in the nut mixture.
5. Transfer the fillets to the baking sheet and brush the fillets with 2 tablespoons olive oil.
6. Place the baking sheet in the preheated oven and bake for 12 to 15 minutes, or until the fish is flaky.
7. Remove from the oven and let cool for 6 minutes before serving.

TIP: You can use the coconut flour for the "breaded" fish fillets before baking.

PER SERVING
calories: 391 | fat: 31.3g | protein: 26.2g | net carbs: 1.1g | fiber: 2g

Ingredients:

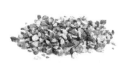

¼ cup almonds, finely chopped

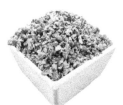

½ cup pecans, finely chopped

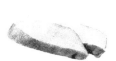

4 (4-ounce / 113-g) boneless halibut fillets, patted dry

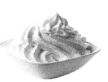

½ cup heavy whipping cream

FROM THE CUPBOARD:

Sea salt and freshly ground black pepper, to taste

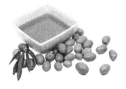

2 tablespoons extra-virgin olive oil

SIMPLE BAKED TROUT WITH SESAME-GINGER DRESSING

Macros: Fat 72% | Protein 26% | Carbs 2%

Prep time: 10 minutes | Cook time: 15 minutes | Serves 4

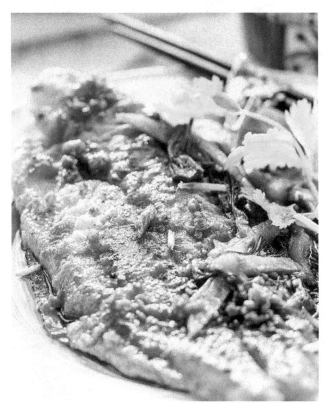

1. Preheat the oven to 400°F (205°C) and grease a baking dish with the olive oil. Set aside.
2. On a clean work surface, lightly sprinkle the fillets with salt and pepper.
3. Transfer the seasoned fillets to the greased baking dish, then drizzle with 1 tablespoon dressing.
4. Place the baking dish in the preheated oven and bake for 12 to 14 minutes, or until the fish flakes easily with a fork.
5. Transfer the fillets to four serving plate and pour the remaining dressing over them. Garnish with the lime wedges and cilantro on top before serving.

TIP: To make this a complete meal, serve it with zucchini noodles.

PER SERVING
calories: 303 | fat: 24.3g | protein: 20.1g | net carbs: 1.1g | fiber: 0g

Ingredients:

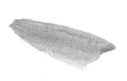

4 (3-ounce / 85-g) trout fillets, patted dry

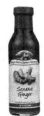

½ cup sesame-ginger dressing

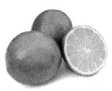

1 quartered lime, for garnish

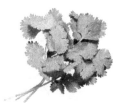

1 tablespoon chopped fresh cilantro, for garnish

FROM THE CUPBOARD:

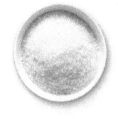

Sea salt and freshly ground black pepper, to taste

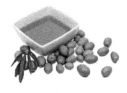

1 tablespoon olive oil, for greasing the baking dish

LOW-CARB THAI FISH WITH BROCCOLI

Macros: Fat 77% | Protein 19% | Carbs 4%

Prep time: 10 minutes | Cook time: 20 minutes | Serves 4

1. Preheat the oven to 400°F (205°C) and lightly grease a baking dish with the olive oil. Set aside.
2. In a bowl, lightly season the fish pieces with salt and pepper.
3. Transfer the fish to the greased baking dish, then brush each fish piece generously with the butter.
4. In a small bowl, stir together the curry paste, coconut cream, and fresh cilantro. Pour this mixture over the fish pieces.
5. Place the baking dish in the preheated oven and bake until the fish is cooked through, about 20 minutes.
6. Meanwhile, add the broccoli florets into a pot of boiling salted water. Allow to boil for 4 to 5 minutes until fork-tender but still crisp. Remove from the heat.
7. Remove the fish from the oven and serve with the broccoli on the side.

TIP: The canned coconut milk can be used as a substitute for coconut cream, but remember use two cans.

PER SERVING
calories: 923 | fat: 79.3g | protein: 42.2g | net carbs: 10.1g | fiber: 5g

Ingredients:

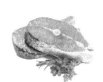

1½ pounds (680 g) salmon or white fish, cut into pieces

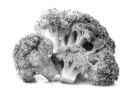

1 pound (454 g) broccoli, cut into florets

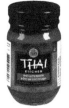

2 tablespoons red curry paste

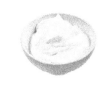

2 cups canned and unsweetened coconut cream

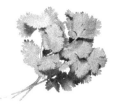

½ cup fresh cilantro, chopped

FROM THE CUPBOARD:

Salt and pepper, to taste

4 tablespoons butter, melted

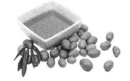

1 tablespoon olive oil, for greasing the baking dish

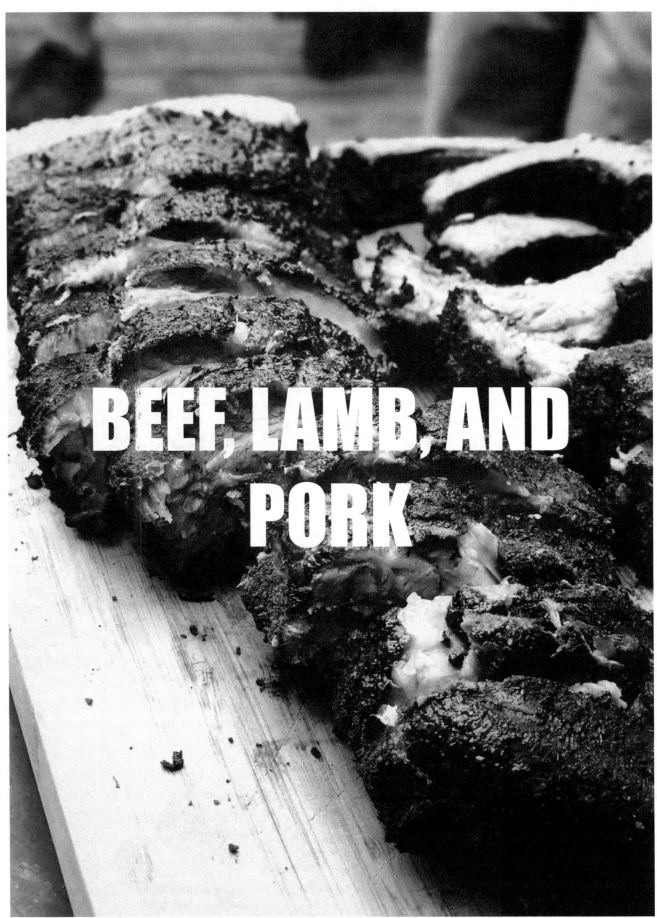

BEEF, LAMB, AND PORK

ITALIAN FLAVOR PORK CHOPS WITH PARSLEY

Macros: Fat 63% | Protein 37% | Carbs 0%

Prep time: 5 minutes | Cook time: 25 minutes | Serves 2

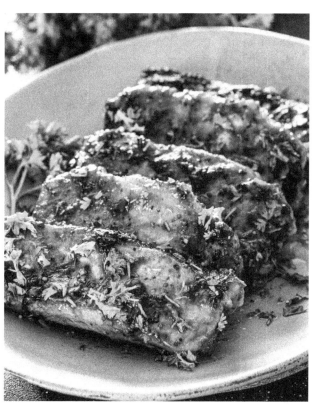

1. Preheat the oven to 350°F (180°C).
2. Coat a baking dish with melted butter. Arrange the pork chops on the dish, then sprinkle with Italian seasoning, salt, and black pepper. Toss to coat well.
3. Spread the chopped parsley over the pork chops, then drizzle them with olive oil and 1 tablespoon butter.
4. Place the baking dish in the preheated oven and bake for about 25 minutes, or until the pork chops are cooked through.
5. Remove the baking dish from the oven, and transfer the pork chops to two platters. Pour the buttery juices remaining on the baking dish over the pork chops before serving.

TIP: To make this a complete meal, you can serve it with mashed cauliflower. They also taste great paired with mushroom and broccoli salad.

PER SERVING
calories: 335 | total fat: 23.5g | total carbs: 0g | fiber: 0g | net carbs: 0g | protein: 30.8g

Ingredients:

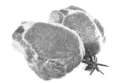

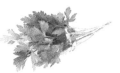

2 boneless pork chops, rinsed and patted dry

1 tablespoon dried Italian seasoning

1 tablespoon chopped fresh flat-leaf Italian parsley

FROM THE CUPBOARD:

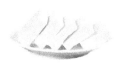

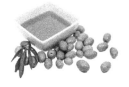

Salt and freshly ground black pepper, to taste

1 tablespoon melted butter, plus more for coating the baking dish

1 tablespoon olive oil

CRUSTED PORK CHOPS WITH ASPARAGUS

Macros: Fat 52% | Protein 43% | Carbs 5%

Prep time: 10 minutes | Cook time: 25 minutes | Serves 2

1. Preheat the oven to 350°F (180°C). Line the aluminum foil on a baking sheet. Set aside.
2. Combine the pork rinds, Parmesan cheese, 1 tablespoon olive oil, and garlic powder in a bowl. Set aside.
3. Place the pork chops in another bowl, then sprinkle salt and black pepper to season. Toss to coat well.
4. Dunk the pork chops in the bowl of pork rind mixture. Arrange the well-coated pork chops on the baking sheet.
5. Arrange the asparagus on the baking sheet beside the pork chops. Drizzle the remaining olive over the asparagus, and sprinkle with the left pork rind mixture, salt, and black pepper.
6. Put the baking sheet in the preheated oven and bake for 25 minutes or until the pork chops are cooked through.
7. Remove the baking sheet from the oven, and transfer the pork chops to two platters, then serve warm.

TIP: To make this a complete meal, you can serve it with garlicky kale salad. They also taste great paired with lemony spinach.

PER SERVING
calories: 372 | total fat: 21.3g | total carbs: 5.9g | fiber: 3.1g | net carbs: 2.8g | protein: 39.7g

Ingredients:

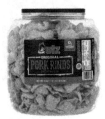
¼ cup crushed pork rinds

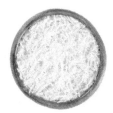
¼ cup grated Parmesan cheese

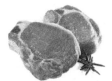
2 boneless pork chops, rinsed and patted dry

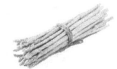
½ pound (227 g) asparagus spears, tough ends snapped off

FROM THE CUPBOARD:

Salt and freshly ground black pepper, to taste

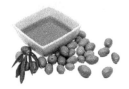
2 tablespoons olive oil

1 teaspoon garlic powder

CARNITAS

Macros: Fat 53% | Protein 40% | Carbs 7%

Prep time: 10 minutes | Cook time: 8 hours | Serves 2

1. Combine the olive oil and chili powder in a bowl. Dunk the pork in the bowl of mixture, then toss to coat well.
2. Arrange the pork in the slow cooker, fat side up. Scatter the diced onion and minced garlic, and sprinkle with salt and black pepper, then drizzle with the lime juice.
3. Put the slow cooker lid on and cook for 8 hours.
4. Remove the pork from the slow cooker and slice to serve.

TIP: To make this a complete meal, the best side dish to serve with this dish is cucumber salad.

PER SERVING
calories: 448 | total fat: 26.2g | total carbs: 5.9g | fiber: 2.1g | net carbs: 3.8g | protein: 44.7g

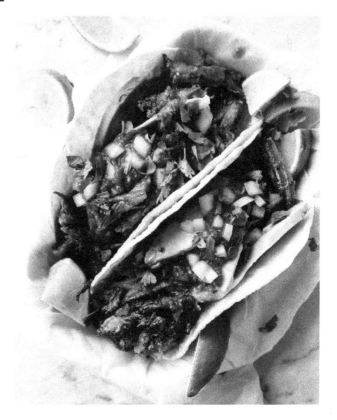

Ingredients:

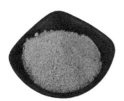

½ tablespoon chili powder

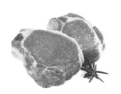

1 pound (454 g) boneless pork butt roast

½ small onion, diced

2 garlic cloves, minced

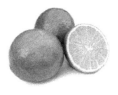

Juice of 1 lime

FROM THE CUPBOARD:

Salt and freshly ground black pepper, to taste

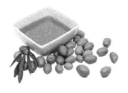

1 tablespoon olive oil

SPECIAL EQUIPMENT:

FRIED STEAKS AND EGGS

Macros: Fat 73% | Protein 26% | Carbs 1%

Prep time: 5 minutes | Cook time: 20 minutes | Serves 2

1. Put the steaks in a bowl, then sprinkle with salt and black pepper. Toss to coat well.
2. In a nonstick skillet, warm 2 tablespoons of olive oil over medium-high heat until shimmering.
3. Add the well-coated steaks to the skillet and fry for 12 minutes or until the steaks are fried through. Flip the steaks halfway through the cooking time. Transfer the steaks to a platter and let stand for at least 10 minutes.
4. Warm the remaining olive oil over medium-low heat in the skillet, then break the eggs in the skillet and fry for 4 minutes or until they reach your desired doneness.
5. Transfer two fried eggs over each steak and top with parsley before serving.

TIP: To make this a complete meal, serve it with a creamy green salad.

PER SERVING
calories: 548 | total fat: 44.2g | total carbs: 1.1g | fiber: 0g | net carbs: 1.1g | protein: 34.8g

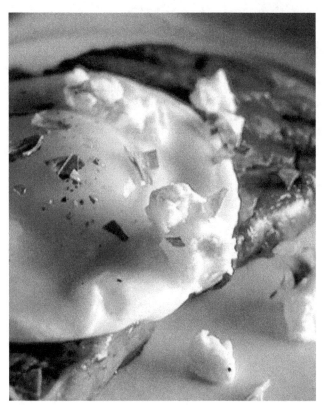

Ingredients:

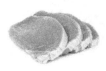

2 (4-ounce / 113-g) strip loin steaks

4 large eggs

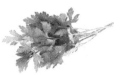

1 teaspoon chopped fresh parsley

FROM THE CUPBOARD:

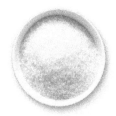

Salt and freshly ground black pepper, to taste

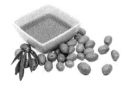

3 tablespoons extra-virgin olive oil, divided

BROILED SIRLOIN STEAK WITH MUSTARD SAUCE

Macros: Fat 78% | Protein 21% | Carbs 1%

Prep time: 10 minutes | Cook time: 15 minutes | Serves 4

1. Preheat the oven to 450°F (235°C).
2. Put the steaks in a bowl, and sprinkle with salt and black pepper. Toss to coat well.
3. Arrange the steaks on a baking sheet, and brush with olive oil on both sides.
4. Place the baking sheet in the preheated oven and broil for 15 minutes or until the steaks are medium-rare. Flip the steaks halfway through the cooking time.
5. Meanwhile, mix the mustard and cream in a saucepan, then bring the mixture to a boil over medium heat to make the sauce.
6. When the sauce is boiling, turn down the heat to low and simmer for 5 minutes or until the sauce reduces about one third.
7. Turn the heat off, then mix in the thyme.
8. Remove the steaks from the oven to four plates, then pour the mustard sauce over the steaks. Let stand for at least 10 minutes and serve warm.

TIP: To make this a complete meal, serve it with salmon, roasted chicken, grilled pork, or green salad.

PER SERVING
calories: 506 | total fat: 43.2g | total carbs: 1.9g | fiber: 0g | net carbs: 1.9g | protein: 24.1g

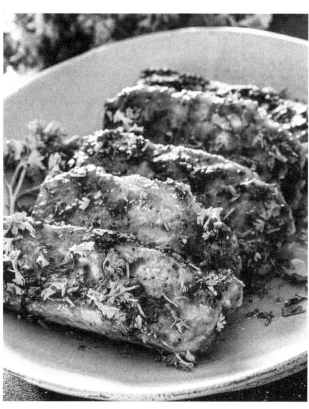

Ingredients:

4 (4-ounce / 113-g) sirloin steaks

MUSHTARD SAUCE:

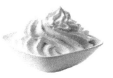

¼ cup grainy mustard

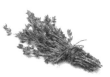

1 cup heavy whipping cream

1 teaspoon chopped fresh thyme

FROM THE CUPBOARD:

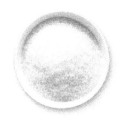

Salt and freshly ground black pepper, to taste

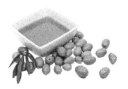

2 tablespoons extra-virgin olive oil

GRILLED STEAKS WITH ANCHOVY BUTTER

Macros: Fat 76% | Protein 24% | Carbs 0%

Prep time: 15 minutes | Cook time: 10 minutes | Serves 4

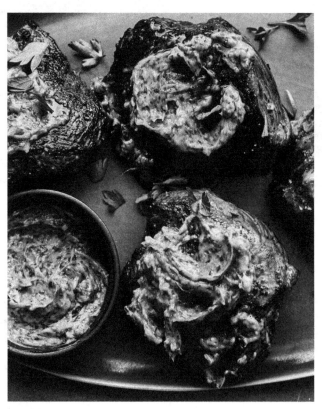

1. Preheat the grill to medium-high heat.
2. Make the anchovy butter: Combine the anchovies, garlic, lemon juice, and butter in a small bowl. Wrap the bowl in plastic and refrigerate to marinate until ready to use.
3. Put the rib eye steaks in a large bowl, and sprinkle with salt and black pepper. Toss to coat well.
4. Brush the grill grates with olive oil. Arrange the steaks on the grill and grill for 10 minutes or until the steaks are medium-rare. Flip the steaks halfway through the cooking time. Brush the steaks with more olive oil as needed during the grilling.
5. Transfer the steaks to four platters and spread the anchovy butter on top before serving.

TIP: To make this a complete meal, serve it with roasted chicken breasts, grilled pork chops, or green salad.

PER SERVING
calories: 448 | total fat: 38.2g | total carbs: 0g | fiber: 0g | net carbs: 0g | protein: 25.8g

Ingredients:

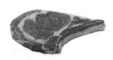

4 (4-ounce / 113-g) rib eye steaks

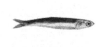

4 anchovies packed in oil, drained and minced

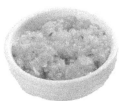

1 teaspoon minced garlic

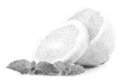

½ teaspoon freshly squeezed lemon juice

FROM THE CUPBOARD:

Salt and freshly ground black pepper, to taste

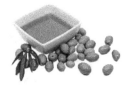

2 tablespoons olive oil, plus more for greasing the grill grates

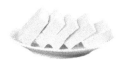

¼ cup unsalted butter, at room temperature

BRIE AND PANCETTA STUFFED PORK TENDERLOIN ROLLS

Macros: Fat 68% | Protein 30% | Carbs 2%

Prep time: 20 minutes | Cook time: 8 hours | Serves 4

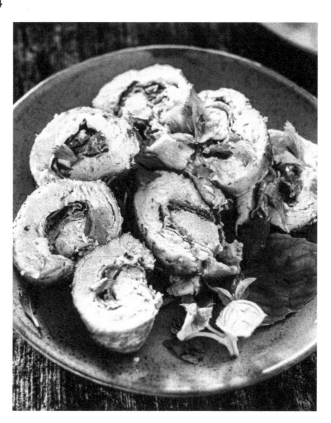

1. Coat the insert of a slow cooker with olive oil.
2. Arrange the pork tenderloins on a clean work surface. Butterfly the tenderloins by cutting them crosswise and leave a 1-inch edge uncut.
3. Open the tenderloins like a book and wrap with plastic. Flatten the tenderloins to ½-inch thick with a rolling pin, then let sit on the work surface.
4. Combine the pancetta, basil, black pepper, garlic, and brie in a bowl. Stir well.
5. Spread the pancetta mixture over the tenderloins, and leave 1-inch edges around the tenderloins.
6. Roll the tenderloins up and run the toothpicks through to secure.
7. Arrange the pork tenderloins in the greased slow cooker and cook on LOW for 8 hours.
8. Remove the tenderloins from the slow cooker, and remove the toothpicks before serving.

TIP: To make this a complete meal, serve it with smoky shredded Brussels sprouts or arugula salad.

PER SERVING
calories: 424 | total fat: 32.1g | total carbs: 1.1g | fiber: 0g | net carbs: 1.1g | protein: 33.8g

Ingredients:

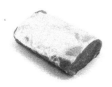

2 (½-pound / 227-g) pork tenderloins

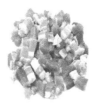

4 ounces (113 g) pancetta, cooked crispy and chopped

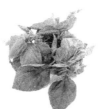

1 teaspoon chopped fresh basil

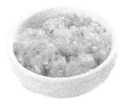

1 teaspoon minced garlic

4 ounces (113 g) triple-cream brie

FROM THE CUPBOARD:

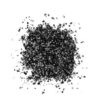

⅛ teaspoon freshly ground black pepper

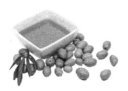

1 tablespoon extra-virgin olive oil

SPECIAL EQUIPMENT:

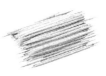

Toothpicks, soak in water for at least 30 minutes

PORK WITH LEMONY CHICKEN BROTH

Macros: Fat 65% | Protein 34% | Carbs 1%

Prep time: 15 minutes | Cook time: 8 hours | Serves 6

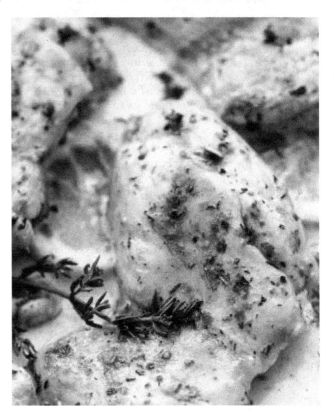

1. Coat the insert of a slow cooker with 1 tablespoon olive oil.
2. Warm the remaining olive oil and melt the butter over medium-high heat in a nonstick skillet.
3. Put the pork in a bowl, and sprinkle with salt and black pepper. Toss to coat well.
4. Place the pork in the skillet and roast for 10 minutes or until well browned. Flip the pork halfway through the cooking time. Arrange the roasted pork in the greased slow cooker.
5. Combine the lemon juice and zest, garlic, and chicken broth in a separate bowl. Pour the mixture over the pork.
6. Put the slow cooker lid on and cook on LOW for 8 hours.
7. Remove the pork from the slow cooker and top with cream before serving.

TIP: To make this a complete meal, serve it with smoky shredded Brussels sprouts or arugula salad.

PER SERVING
calories: 449 | total fat: 31.2g | total carbs: 1.1g | fiber: 0g | net carbs: 1.1g | protein: 38.8g

Ingredients:

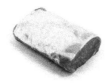

2 pounds (907 g) pork loin roast

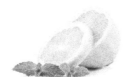

Juice and zest of 1 lemon

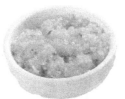

1 tablespoon minced garlic

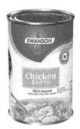

¼ cup chicken broth

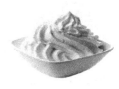

½ cup heavy whipping cream

FROM THE CUPBOARD:

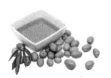

3 tablespoons extra-virgin olive oil, divided

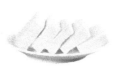

1 tablespoon butter

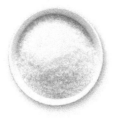

½ teaspoon salt

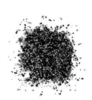

¼ teaspoon freshly ground black pepper

PORK IN BACON ROLLS

Macros: Fat 73% | Protein 26% | Carbs 1%

Prep time: 15 minutes | Cook time: 6 hours | Serves 8

1. Coat the insert of a slow cooker with 1 tablespoon olive oil.
2. Put the pork in a large bowl, and sprinkle with onion power, garlic powder, salt, and black pepper. Toss to coat well.
3. Warm the remaining olive oil in a nonstick skillet over medium-high heat until shimmering.
4. Place the pork in the skillet and roast for 10 minutes or until well browned. Flip the pork halfway through the cooking time. Allow to cool for 10 minutes.
5. Wrap the bacon slices around the pork, securing with a toothpick. Place them in the greased slow cooker, and add the thyme, oregano, and chicken broth.
6. Put the slow cooker lid on and cook on LOW for 6 hours.
7. Remove the pork from the slow cooker and serve warm.

TIP: To make this a complete meal, serve it with roasted broccoli or Balsamic sauced Brussels sprouts.

PER SERVING
calories: 494 | total fat: 40.2g | total carbs: 1.1g | fiber: 0g | net carbs: 1.1g | protein: 30.8g

Ingredients:

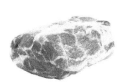

2 pounds (907 g) pork shoulder roast

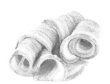

8 bacon strips

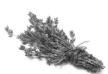

2 teaspoons chopped thyme

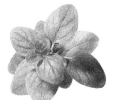

1 teaspoon chopped oregano

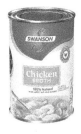

¼ cup chicken broth

FROM THE CUPBOARD: SPECIAL EQUIPMENT:

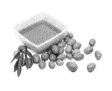

3 tablespoons extra-virgin olive oil, divided

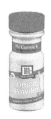

1 teaspoon onion powder

1 teaspoon garlic powder

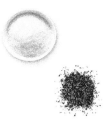

Salt and freshly ground black pepper, to taste

Toothpicks, sock in water for at least 30 minutes

ROAST BEEF WITH KETCHUP AND CIDER BROTH

Macros: Fat 73% | Protein 24% | Carbs 3%

Prep time: 15 minutes | Cook time: 9 hours | Serves 8

1. Coat the insert of a slow cooker with 1 tablespoon olive oil.
2. Put the beef in a large bowl, and sprinkle with salt and black pepper. Toss to coat well.
3. Warm the remaining olive oil in a nonstick skillet over medium-high heat until shimmering.
4. Place the beef in the skillet and cook for 6 minutes or until well browned. Flip the beef halfway through the cooking time. Transfer the cooked beef into the greased slow cooker.
5. Combine the ketchup, apple cider vinegar, ginger, and beef broth in a separate bowl. Stir well. Pour the mixture over the beef in the slow cooker.
6. Put the slow cooker lid on and cook on LOW for 9 hours.
7. Remove the beef from the slow cooker and serve warm.

TIP: To make this a complete meal, serve it with roasted broccoli or Balsamic sauced Brussels sprouts.

PER SERVING
calories: 483 | total fat: 39.1g | total carbs: 3.8g | fiber: 0g | net carbs: 3.8g | protein: 28.8g

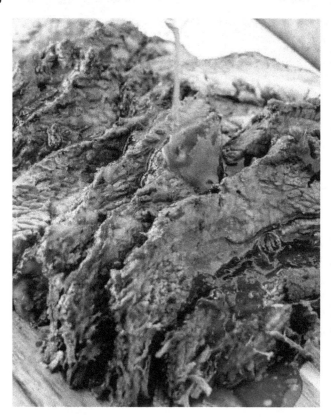

Ingredients:

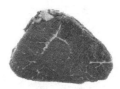

2 pounds (907 g) beef boneless chuck roast

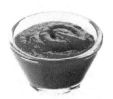

¼ cup low-carb ketchup

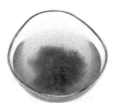

2 tablespoons apple cider vinegar

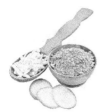

2 tablespoons grated fresh ginger

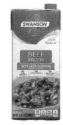

½ cup beef broth

FROM THE CUPBOARD:

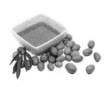

⅛ teaspoon freshly ground black pepper

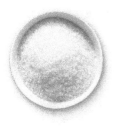

½ teaspoon salt

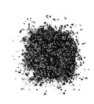

¼ cup extra-virgin olive oil, divided

68   Beef, Lamb, And Pork

GARLICKY LAMB LEG WITH STOCK AND DRY RED WINE

Macros: Fat 36% | Protein 62% | Carbs 2%

Prep time: 15 minutes | Cook time: 10 hours | Serves 8

1. Coat the insert of a slow cooker with 1 tablespoon olive oil.
2. Warm the remaining olive oil in a nonstick skillet over medium-high heat until shimmering.
3. Put the lamb leg in a large bowl, and sprinkle with salt and black pepper. Toss to coat well.
4. Put the lamb leg in the skillet and sear for 2 minutes or until well browned. Flip the lamb leg halfway through the cooking time. Set aside.
5. Add the stock and dry red wine to the skillet and simmer to lightly thicken the mixture. Keep stirring during the simmering. Turn off the heat and let sit until ready to use.
6. Make 12 slits on the lamb leg with a knife, then press the halves of garlic clove into each slit. Spread the top of the lamb leg with Dijon mustard.
7. Arrange the lamb leg in the greased slow cooker, then pour over the stick and dry red wine mixture.
8. Put the slow cooker lid on and cook on LOW for 10 hours.
9. Remove the lamb leg from the slow cooker. Allow to cook for 30 minutes, then slice to serve.

TIP: To make this a complete meal, serve it with roasted butternut squash.

PER SERVING
calories: 318 | total fat: 12.2g | total carbs: 1.4g | fiber: 0g | net carbs: 1.4g | protein: 46.7g

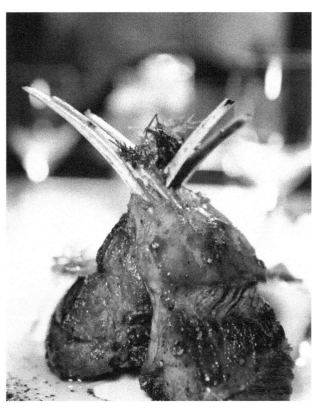

Ingredients:

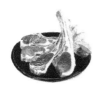

4 pounds (113 g) leg of lamb, bone in

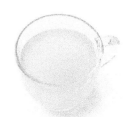

1 cup lamb or beef stock

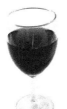

¾ cup dry red wine

6 garlic cloves, cut in half

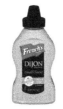

2 tablespoons Dijon mustard

FROM THE CUPBOARD:

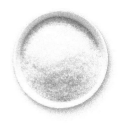

Salt and freshly ground black pepper, to taste

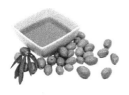

¼ cup extra-virgin olive oil, divided

BRAISED LAMB

Macros: Fat 41% | Protein 54% | Carbs 5%

Prep time: 10 minutes | Cook time: 5 minutes | Serves 4

1. Heat the olive oil over medium-high heat in a nonstick skillet until shimmering.
2. Put the lamb chops in a large bowl, and sprinkle with salt and black pepper. Toss to coat well.
3. Put the lamb chops in the skillet and sauté for 2 minutes or until well browned. Flip the lamb chops halfway through the cooking time. Set aside.
4. Add the tomato sauce and onion to the skillet and cook for 2 minutes or until the onion is translucent, then mix in the broth.
5. Place the lamb chops and the tomato sauce mixture in a pressure cooker. Put the lid on and cook for 2 minutes.
6. Release the pressure and transfer the lamb and sauce to a large platter to serve.

TIP: To make this a complete meal, serve it with roasted courgette.

PER SERVING
calories: 352 | total fat: 16.2g | total carbs: 2.4g | fiber: 0g | net carbs: 2.4g | protein: 47.4g

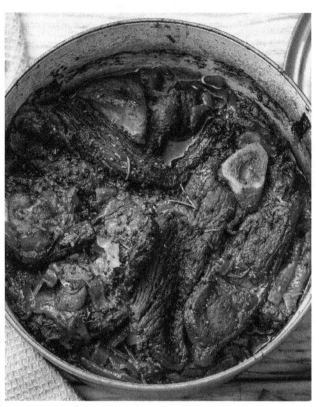

Ingredients:

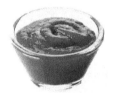

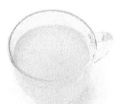

| 8 bone-in lamb chops (about 2 pounds / 907 g) | ¼ cup low-carb tomato sauce | 1 small yellow onion, diced | 1 cup lamb or beef broth |

FROM THE CUPBOARD:

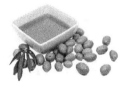

Salt and freshly ground black pepper, to taste   1 tablespoon olive oil

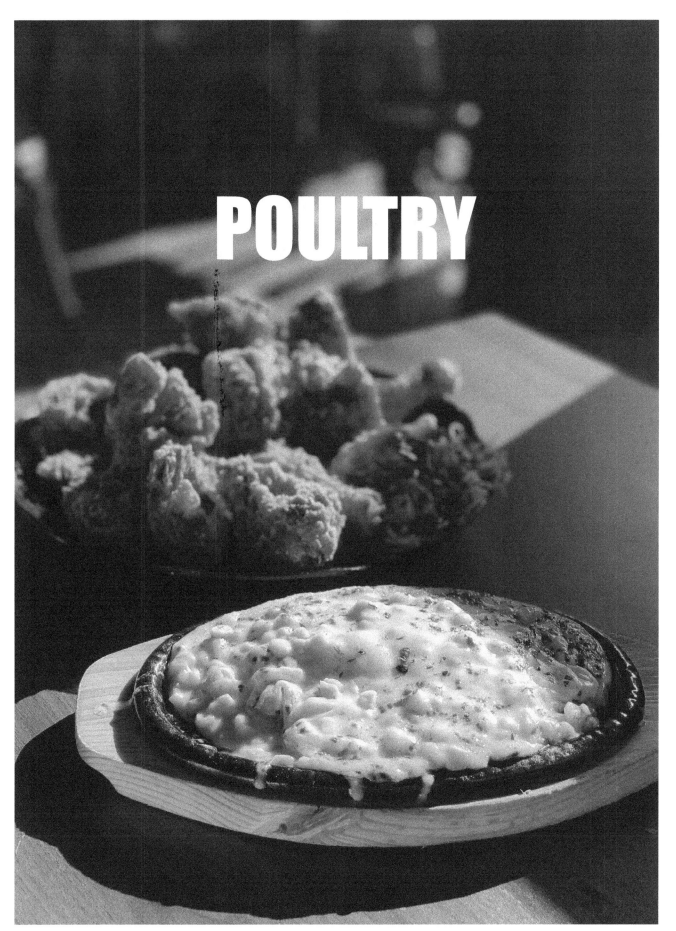

POULTRY

CRISPY CRUSTED CHICKEN WINGS

Macros: Fat 79% | Protein 19% | Carbs 2%

Prep time: 10 minutes | Cook time: 3 hours | Serves 2

1. Line the aluminum foil on a baking sheet.
2. Add the Italian seasoning, ¼ cup of Parmesan cheese, garlic, butter, salt, and black pepper to the slow cooker. Blend to combine well.
3. Put the chicken wings into the slow cooker, then stir to coat the wings well.
4. Put the slow cooker lid on and cook on HIGH for 2 hours and 45 minutes.
5. Preheat the oven to 400°F (205°C).
6. Remove the chicken wings from the slow cooker to the baking sheet, then spread the remaining Parmesan cheese over the wings.
7. Put the baking sheet in the preheated oven and cook for 5 minutes or until the wings are crispy.
8. Transfer the chicken wings to a platter and serve hot.

TIP: To make this a complete meal, you can serve it with mashed cauliflower. They also taste great paired with mushroom and spinach salad.

PER SERVING
calories: 739 | total fat: 64.8g | total carbs: 3.9g | fiber: 0g | net carbs: 3.9g | protein: 36.2g

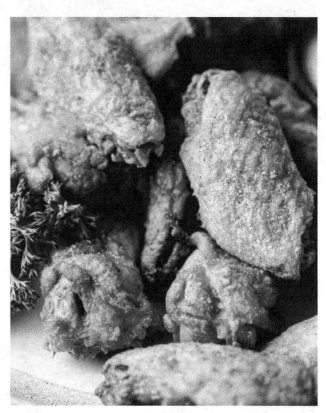

Ingredients:

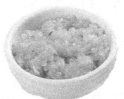

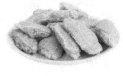

1 tablespoon dried Italian seasoning

¼ cup grated Parmesan cheese, plus ½ cup

2 garlic cloves, minced

1 pound (454 g) chicken wings

FROM THE CUPBOARD:

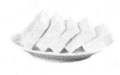

Salt and freshly ground black pepper, to taste

8 tablespoons (1 stick) butter

LEMONY CHICKEN THIGHS WITH KALAMATA OLIVES

Macros: Fat 75% | Protein 23% | Carbs 2%

Prep time: 10 minutes | Cook time: 40 minutes | Serves 2

1. Preheat the oven to 375°F (190°C).
2. Put the chicken thighs in a large bowl, then sprinkle with salt and black pepper. Toss to coat well.
3. Melt the ghee over medium-high heat in a oven-safe skillet, then put the chicken thighs in the skillet, skin side down.
4. Cook for 8 minutes or until the skin is crisp and well browned, then turn the thighs over and cook for 2 minutes more.
5. After cooking, pour the chicken broth over the thighs, add the olives and sliced lemon, and squeeze the lemon juice over.
6. Arrange the skillet in the preheated oven and bake for 30 minutes or until an instant-read thermometer inserted in the center of the thigh registers at least 165°F (74°C).
7. Remove the skillet from the oven. Drizzle the butter over the broth mixture, then serve them warm in a large platter.

TIP: To make this a complete meal, you can serve it with creamed spinach. They also taste great paired with tomato and zucchini casserole.

PER SERVING
calories: 568 | total fat: 47.2g | total carbs: 3.4g | fiber: 2.1g | net carbs: 1.3g | protein: 32.8g

Ingredients:

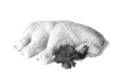

4 chicken thighs, rinsed and patted dry

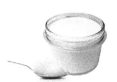

2 tablespoons ghee

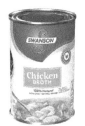

½ cup chicken broth

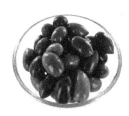

½ cup pitted Kalamata olives

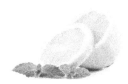

1 lemon, ½ sliced and ½ juiced

FROM THE CUPBOARD:

SPECIAL EQUIPMENT:

Salt and freshly ground black pepper, to taste

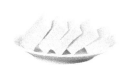

2 tablespoons melted butter

TOMATO AND PECAN STUFFED CHICKEN THIGHS

Macros: Fat 77% | Protein 20% | Carbs 3%

Prep time: 20 minutes | Cook time: 30 minutes | Serves 4

1. Preheat the oven to 350°F (180°C).
2. Combine the tomatoes, pecans, and goat cheese in a bowl.
3. Loose the skin on each chicken thigh to form a pocket with your fingers.
4. Spoon the tomato mixture in the pocket gently, then cover the mixture with the skin.
5. In an oven-safe skillet, warm the olive oil over medium-high heat. Put the chicken thighs in the skillet, skin side down, and season with salt and black pepper.
6. Sear for 8 minutes or until the skin is crisp and well browned, then turn the thighs over and sear for 2 minutes more.
7. Pour the chicken broth over the thighs, then cover the skillet with aluminum foil and arrange in the preheated oven.
8. Bake for 20 minutes or until an instant-read thermometer inserted in the center of the thigh registers at least 165°F (74°C).
9. Remove them from the oven and divide to four plates, then serve warm.

TIP: To make this a complete meal, you can serve it with creamed spinach. They also taste great paired with tomato and zucchini casserole.

PER SERVING
calories: 556 | total fat: 48.2g | total carbs: 3.3g | fiber: 2.1g | net carbs: 1.2g | protein: 27.8g

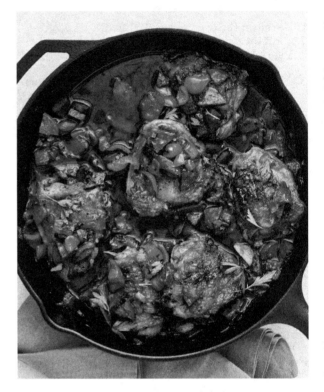

Ingredients:

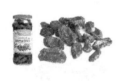

2 tablespoons chopped sun-dried tomatoes

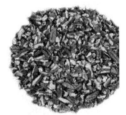

½ cup chopped pecans

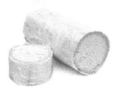

4 ounces (113 g) goat cheese

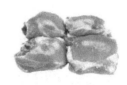

4 (5-ounce / 142-g) skin-on, boneless chicken thighs, rinsed and patted dry

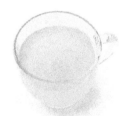

¼ cup low-sodium chicken broth

FROM THE CUPBOARD:

Salt and freshly ground black pepper, to taste

SPECIAL EQUIPMENT:

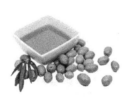

2 tablespoons extra-virgin olive oil

CHEESY SPINACH AND PEPPERS WITH GRILLED CHICKEN

Macros: Fat 44% | Protein 52% | Carbs 4%

Prep time: 10 minutes | Cook time: 25 minutes | Serves 6

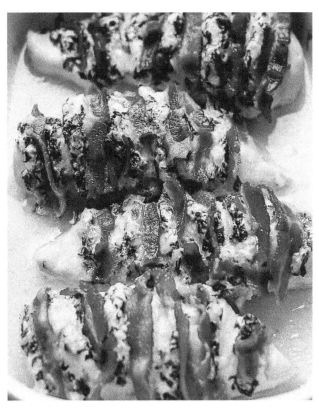

1. Preheat the oven to 400°F (205°C). Grease a baking pan with 1 tablespoon olive oil.
2. Heat 1 tablespoon of the olive oil in a nonstick skillet, then put the chicken breasts in the skillet. Sprinkle with salt and black pepper, and cook for 6 minutes or until well browned. Flip the breasts halfway through the cooking time. Set the cooked chicken breasts aside.
3. Heat the remaining olive oil in the skillet and add the spinach and garlic to the skillet. Sprinkle with salt and black pepper, and cook for 3 minutes or until the spinach is tender.
4. Arrange the cooked chicken in the greased baking pan, then add the spinach and garlic, mozzarella cheese, and roasted peppers.
5. Bake in the preheated oven for 15 minutes or until an instant-read thermometer inserted in the center of the thigh registers at least 165°F (74°C).
6. Remove the baking pan from the oven, then serve them warm in a large plate.

TIP: To make this a complete meal, you can serve it with cheesy baked asparagus. They also taste great paired with cucumber salad.

PER SERVING
calories: 292 | total fat: 14.4g | total carbs: 3.3g | fiber: 2.1g | net carbs: 1.2g | protein: 36.2g

Ingredients:

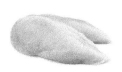

3 large chicken breasts, sliced in Half

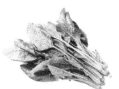

10 ounces (284 g) spinach, frozen, thawed, and blanched

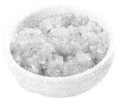

2 cloves garlic, minced

3 ounces (85 g) mozzarella cheese, shredded

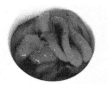

½ cup roasted red peppers, sliced into strips

FROM THE CUPBOARD:

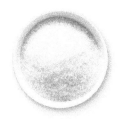

Salt and freshly ground black pepper, to taste

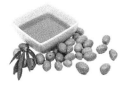

3 tablespoons olive oil, divided

TURKEY AND SWEET ONION MEATLOAF

Macros: Fat 69% | Protein 29% | Carbs 2%

Prep time: 10 minutes | Cook time: 35 minutes | Serves 6

1. Preheat the oven to 450°F (235°C).
2. Warm the olive oil over medium heat in a nonstick skillet.
3. Add and sauté the onion for 4 minutes or until translucent.
4. Put the cooked onion in a large bowl, then add the ground turkey, cheese, parsley, cream, salt, and black pepper. Stir to combine well.
5. Press the mixture into a loaf pan, then place in the preheated oven and bake for 30 minutes or until cooked through.
6. Transfer the meatloaf to a serving pan and allow to cool for 10 minutes before serving.

TIP: To make this a complete meal, you can serve it with cheesy baked asparagus. They also taste great paired with cucumber salad.

PER SERVING
calories: 218 | total fat: 19.2g | total carbs: 1g | fiber: 0g | net carbs: 1g | protein: 14.8g

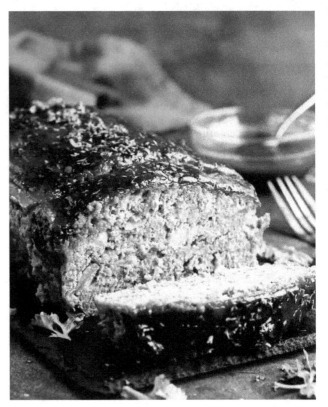

Ingredients:

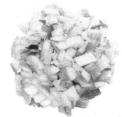

½ sweet onion, chopped

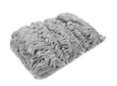

1½ pounds (680 g) ground turkey

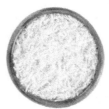

¼ cup freshly grated Parmesan cheese

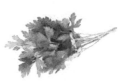

1 tablespoon chopped fresh parsley

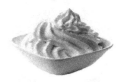

⅓ cup heavy whipping cream

FROM THE CUPBOARD:

Salt and freshly ground black pepper, to taste

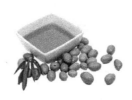

1 tablespoon olive oil

SPECIAL EQUIPMENT:

CHEESY BACON-WRAPPED CHICKEN WITH ASPARAGUS SPEARS

Macros: Fat 75% | Protein 23% | Carbs 2%

Prep time: 20 minutes | Cook time: 30 minutes | Serves 4

1. Preheat the oven to 400°F (205°C). Line a baking sheet with parchment paper, then grease with 1 tablespoon olive oil.
2. Put the chicken breasts in a large bowl, and sprinkle with salt and black pepper. Toss to combine well.
3. Wrap each chicken breast with 2 slices of bacon. Place the chicken on the baking sheet, then bake in the preheated oven for 25 minutes or until the bacon is crispy.
4. Preheat the grill to high, then brush with the remaining olive oil.
5. Place the asparagus spears on the grill grate, and sprinkle with salt. Grill for 5 minutes or until fork-tender. Flip the asparagus frequently during the grilling.
6. Transfer the bacon-wrapped chicken breasts to four plates, drizzle with lemon juice, and scatter with Manchego cheese. Spread the hot asparagus spears on top to serve.

TIP: To make this a complete meal, you can serve it with mashed cauliflower.

PER SERVING
calories: 455 | total fat: 38.1g | net carbs: 2g | protein: 26.1g

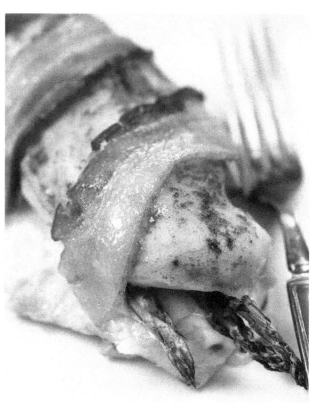

Ingredients:

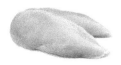

4 chicken breasts

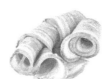

8 bacon slices

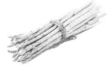

1 pound (454 g) asparagus spears

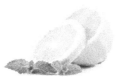

2 tablespoons fresh lemon juice

½ cup Manchego cheese, grated

FROM THE CUPBOARD:

Salt and freshly ground black pepper, to taste

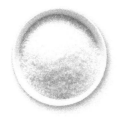

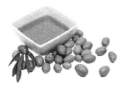

4 tablespoons olive oil, divided

ALMOND CRUSTED CHICKEN

Macros: Fat 65% | Protein 35% | Carbs 0%

Prep time: 10 minutes | Cook time: 15 minutes | Serves 4

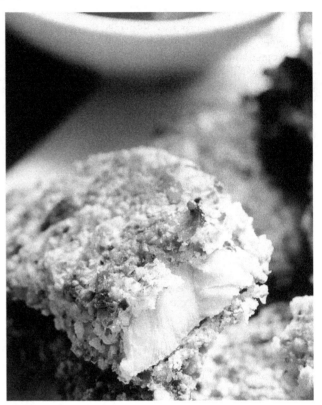

1. Combine the eggs and garlic powder in a bowl.
2. Combine the almond flour and oregano in another bowl.
3. Dunk the chicken breasts in the egg mixture, then in the flour mixture to coat well. Shake the excess off.
4. Heat the olive oil and melt the butter in a nonstick skillet over medium-high heat.
5. Put the well-coated chicken breasts in the skillet. Sprinkle with salt and black pepper, and fry for 14 minutes or until crispy. Flip the chicken breasts halfway through the cooking time.
6. Remove the breasts from the skillet to four plates and serve warm.

TIP: To make this a complete meal, you can serve it with cheesy zucchini bake.

PER SERVING
calories: 329 | total fat: 23.2g | total carbs: 0g | fiber: 0g | net carbs: 0g | protein: 27.9g

Ingredients:

2 eggs, whisked

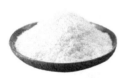

1 cup almond flour

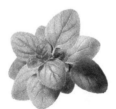

1 tablespoon chopped fresh oregano

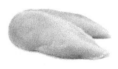

4 (4-ounce / 113-g) boneless skinless chicken breasts, pounded to about ¼-inch thick

FROM THE CUPBOARD:

Salt and freshly ground black pepper, to taste

½ teaspoon garlic powder

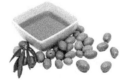

¼ cup olive oil

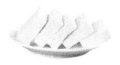

2 tablespoons butter

SPICY CHICKEN BREASTS

Macros: Fat 74% | Protein 25% | Carbs 1%

Prep time: 10 minutes | Cook time: 6 hours | Serves 4

1. Use 1 tablespoon of olive oil to coat the insert of the slow cooker.
2. Warm the remaining olive oil over medium-high heat in a nonstick skillet.
3. Put the chicken breasts in the skillet. Season with salt and black pepper, and cook for 5 minutes or until well browned. Flip the chicken halfway through the cooking time.
4. Arrange the cooked chicken breasts in a singer layer in the slow cooker.
5. Combine the onion, garlic, hot sauce, coconut oil, and water in a bowl, then pour them over the chicken breasts.
6. Put the slow cooker lid on and cook on LOW for 6 hours.
7. Transfer the chicken breasts to four plates and spread the parsley on top before serving.

TIP: To make this a complete meal, you can serve it with cheesy zucchini bake or Parmesan roasted cauliflower.

PER SERVING
calories: 378 | total fat: 31.2g | total carbs: 2g | fiber: 1g | net carbs: 1g | protein: 26.1g

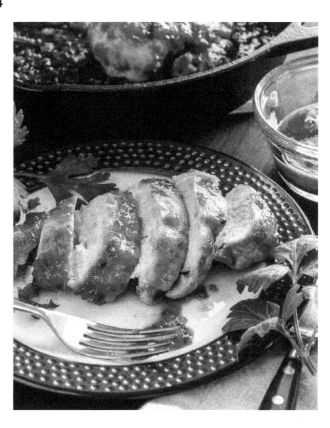

Ingredients:

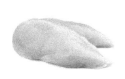

1 pound (454 g) boneless chicken breasts

½ sweet onion, finely chopped

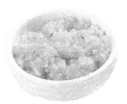

1 teaspoon minced garlic

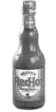

1 cup hot sauce

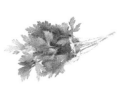

2 tablespoons chopped fresh parsley, for garnishing

FROM THE CUPBOARD:

Salt and freshly ground black pepper, to taste

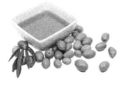

3 tablespoons olive oil, divided

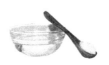

⅓ cup coconut oil, melted

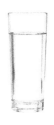

¼ cup water

TURKEY LEGS WITH THYME

Macros: Fat 70% | Protein 29% | Carbs 1%

Prep time: 15 minutes | Cook time: 7 hours | Serves 6

1. Use 1 tablespoon of olive oil to coat the insert of the slow cooker.
2. Warm the remaining olive oil over medium-high heat in a nonstick skillet.
3. Put the turkey legs in a large bowl, then sprinkle with poultry seasoning, thyme, salt, and black pepper. Toss to coat well.
4. Arrange the turkey legs in the skillet and cook for 7 minutes or until well browned. Flip the legs halfway through the cooking time.
5. Place the turkey legs in the slow cooker, then pour the chicken broth over.
6. Put the slow cooker lid on and cook on LOW for 7 hours.
7. Transfer the turkey legs to a large plate and spread the parsley on top before serving.

TIP: To make this a complete meal, you can serve it with cheesy zucchini bake or Parmesan roasted cauliflower.

PER SERVING
calories: 365 | total fat: 29.2g | total carbs: 1g | fiber: 0g | net carbs: 1g | protein: 27.7g

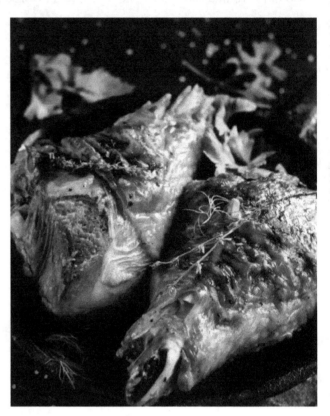

Ingredients:

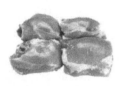

2 pounds (907 g) boneless turkey legs

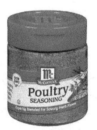

2 teaspoons poultry seasoning

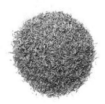

1 tablespoon dried thyme

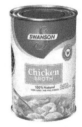

½ cup chicken broth

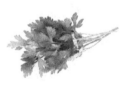

2 tablespoons chopped fresh parsley, for garnishing

FROM THE CUPBOARD:

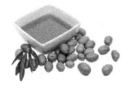

Salt and freshly ground black pepper, to taste

3 tablespoons extra-virgin olive oil, divided

CHICKEN WINGS WITH BUFFALO HOT SAUCE

Macros: Fat 75% | Protein 25% | Carbs 0%

Prep time: 10 minutes | Cook time: 6 hours | Serves 8

1. Grease the insert of the slow cooker with olive oil.
2. Arrange the chicken wing sections in a singer layer in the slow cooker, then season with salt and black pepper.
3. Combine the buffalo bot sauce, onion power, garlic power, oregano, and butter in a bowl, then pour them over the chicken breasts.
4. Put the slow cooker lid on and cook on LOW for 6 hours.
5. Transfer the chicken wing sections to a large platter and serve warm.

TIP: To make this a complete meal, you can serve it with riced cauliflower or roasted Brussels sprouts with bacon.

PER SERVING
calories: 534 | total fat: 44.3g | total carbs: 1g | fiber: 0g | net carbs: 1g | protein: 31.2g

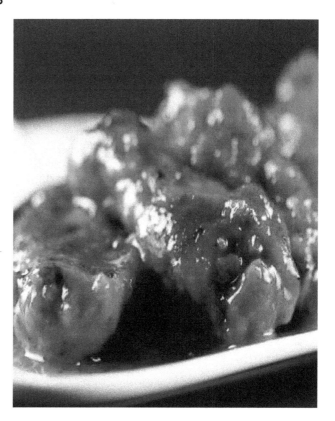

Ingredients:

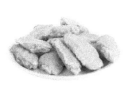

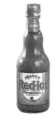

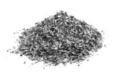

| 3 pounds (1.4 kg) chicken wing sections | 1 (12-ounce / 340-g) bottle buffalo hot sauce | 1 tablespoon dried oregano |

FROM THE CUPBOARD:

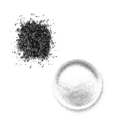

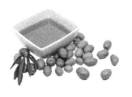

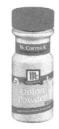

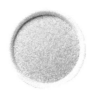

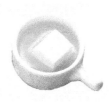

Salt and freshly ground black pepper, to taste

1 tablespoon olive oil

1 teaspoon onion powder

2 teaspoons garlic powder

¾ cup melted butter

BACON-WRAPPED CHICKEN WITH CHEDDAR CHEESE

Macros: Fat 61% | Protein 35% | Carbs 4%

Prep time: 10 minutes | Cook time: 4 hours | Serves 6

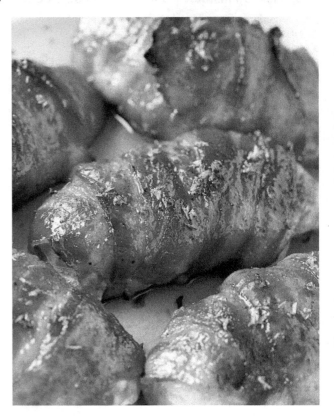

1. Grease the insert of the slow cooker with olive oil.
2. Wrap each piece of chicken breast with each half of bacon slice, and arrange them in the slow cooker. Sprinkle with garlic, salt, and black pepper.
3. Put the slow cooker lid on and cook on LOW for 4 hours.
4. Preheat the oven to 350°F (180°C).
5. Transfer the cooked bacon-wrapped chicken to a baking dish, then scatter with cheese.
6. Cook in the preheated oven for 5 minutes or until the cheese melts.
7. Remove them from the oven and serve warm.

TIP: To make this a complete meal, you can serve it with riced cauliflower or roasted Brussels sprouts with bacon.

PER SERVING
calories: 308 | total fat: 20.8g | total carbs: 2.9g | fiber: 0g | net carbs: 2.9g | protein: 26.1g

Ingredients:

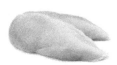

2 large chicken breasts, each cut into 6 pieces

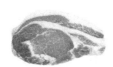

6 slices of streaky bacon, each cut in half width ways

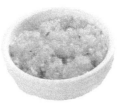

4 garlic cloves, crushed

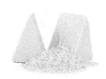

½ cup Cheddar cheese, grated

FROM THE CUPBOARD:

Salt and freshly ground black pepper, to taste

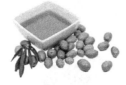

1 tablespoon olive oil

MACADAMIA ENCRUSTED CHICKEN NIBBLES

Macros: Fat 71% | Protein 25% | Carbs 4%

Prep time: 10 minutes | Cook time: 2 hours | Serves 4

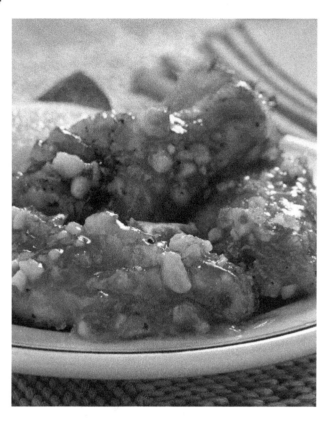

1. Put the macadamia nuts in a bowl, and sprinkle with mixed spices, salt, and black pepper. Stir to mix well.
2. Whisk the eggs in a separate bowl. Dredge the chicken nibbles in the whisked eggs, then in the bowl of macadamia mixture.
3. Grease the insert of the slow cooker with 2 tablespoons of olive oil.
4. Arrange the well-coated chicken nibbles in a singer layer in the slow cooker.
5. Put the slow cooker lid on and cook on HIGH for 2 hours. Flip the chicken nibbles halfway through the cooking time.
6. Warm the remaining olive oil in a nonstick skillet. Put the cooked chicken nibbles in the skillet and fry for 2 minutes on each side or until lightly browned.
7. Transfer the chicken nibbles to a large plate and serve warm.

TIP: To make this a complete meal, you can serve it with homemade garlic aioli and cheesy baked asparagus.

PER SERVING
calories: 319 | total fat: 25.9g | total carbs: 3.1g | fiber: 1.6g | net carbs: 1.5g | protein: 19.1g

Ingredients:

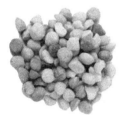

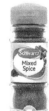

½ cup roasted macadamia nuts, finely chopped

2 teaspoons dried mixed spices (homemade or store-bought)

2 eggs

1.5 pounds (680 g) chicken nibbles

FROM THE CUPBOARD:

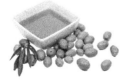

Salt and freshly ground black pepper, to taste

3 tablespoons olive oil, divided

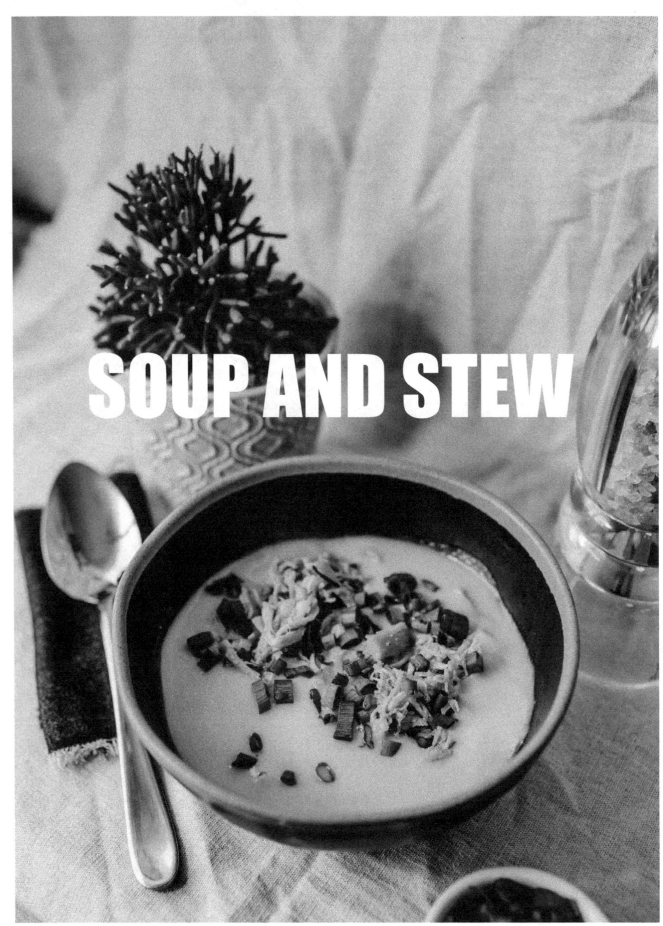

SOUP AND STEW

TOMATO AND BASIL SOUP

Macros: Fat 84% | Protein 5% | Carbs 11%

Prep time: 5 minutes | Cook time: 15 minutes | Serves 4

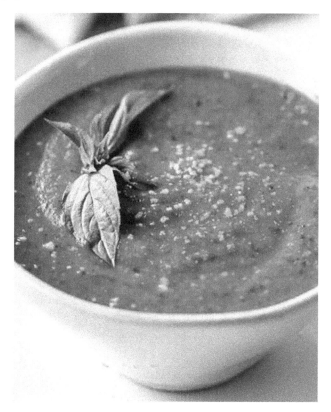

1. Arrange the diced tomatoes in a food processor. Process until smooth.
2. Melt the butter in a saucepan over medium heat. Add the tomato purée, cream, and cheese. Cook for 10 minutes or until well combined. Keep stirring during the cooking.
3. Sprinkle with chopped basil leaves, salt, and black pepper. Keep cooking for an additional 5 minutes or until smooth and the soup has thickened. Stir constantly.
4. Spoon the soup into a large bowl and serve warm.

TIP: To make this a complete meal, you can serve this dish with roasted chicken thighs and a green salad you like.

PER SERVING
calories: 238 | total fat: 22.1g | total carbs: 8.9g | fiber: 2.1g | net carbs: 6.8g | protein: 3.1g

Ingredients:

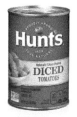

1 (14.5-ounce / 411-g) can diced tomatoes

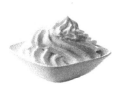

¼ cup heavy whipping cream

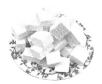

2 ounces (57 g) cream cheese

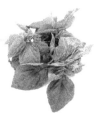

¼ cup chopped fresh basil leaves

FROM THE CUPBOARD:

Salt and freshly ground black pepper, to taste

4 tablespoons butter

CHEESY BROCCOLI SOUP

Macros: Fat 87% | Protein 10% | Carbs 3%

Prep time: 5 minutes | Cook time: 20 minutes | Serves 4

1. Put the butter in a saucepan, and melt over medium heat.
2. Add and sauté the broccoli for 4 to 5 minutes or until soft.
3. Mix in the chicken broth and heavy whipping cream over the broccoli, and sprinkle with salt and black pepper. Cook for about 15 minutes or until the soup is smooth and thickened. Keep stirring during the cooking.
4. Reduce the heat to low and gently fold in the Cheddar cheese. Keep stirring until well combined.
5. Spoon the soup into a large bowl. Scatter more cheese over the soup before serving.

TIP: To make this a complete meal, you can serve this dish with pork chop and a mushroom salad.

PER SERVING
calories: 386 | total fat: 37.3g | total carbs: 3.8g | fiber: 1.1g | net carbs: 2.7g | protein: 9.8g

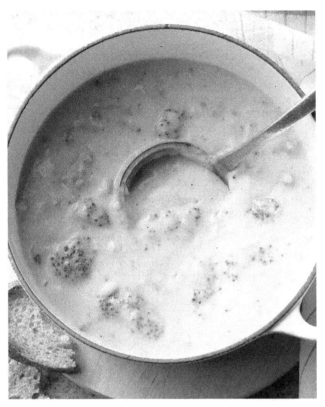

Ingredients:

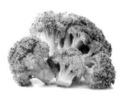

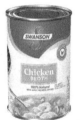

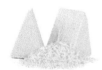

| 1 cup broccoli, cut into florets | 1 cup chicken broth | 1 cup heavy whipping cream | 1 cup shredded Cheddar cheese, plus more for topping |

FROM THE CUPBOARD:

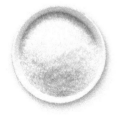

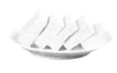

Salt and freshly ground black pepper, to taste

2 tablespoons butter

CAULIFLOWER, COCONUT MILK, AND SHRIMP SOUP

Macros: Fat 72% | Protein 24% | Carbs 4%

Prep time: 5 minutes | Cook time: 2 hours 15 minutes | Serves 4

1. Add the riced cauliflower, red curry paste, coconut milk, 1 tablespoon cilantro, water, then sprinkle with salt and black pepper. Blend the mixture to combine well.
2. Put the slow cooker lid on and cook on HIGH for 2 hours.
3. Put the shrimp on a clean working surface, then sprinkle salt and black pepper to season.
4. Put the shrimp in the slow cooker and cook for 15 minutes more.
5. Transfer the soup into a large bowl and top with the remaining cilantro leaves before serving.

TIP: You can try this recipe with other ingredients, such as replacing the shrimp to chicken breasts, and it will give this recipe a different flavor.

PER SERVING
calories: 268 | total fat: 21.3g | total carbs: 7.8g | fiber: 3.2g | net carbs: 4.6g | protein: 16.1g

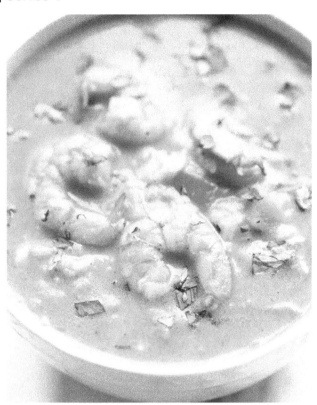

Ingredients:

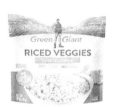
2 cups riced cauliflower

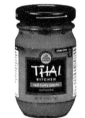
2 tablespoons red curry paste

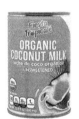
1 (13.5-ounce / 383-g) can unsweetened full-fat coconut milk

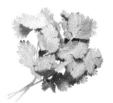
2 tablespoons chopped fresh cilantro leaves, divided

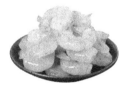
1 cup shrimp, peeled, deveined, tail off, and cooked

FROM THE CUPBOARD:

Salt and freshly ground black pepper, to taste

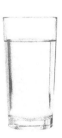
1 cup water

LAMB STEW

Macros: Fat 34% | Protein 59% | Carbs 7%

Prep time: 5 minutes | Cook time: 8 hours | Serves 6

1. Arrange the lamb into a lightly greased nonstick skillet, and cook over high heat for 2 minutes or until browned.
2. Grease a slow cooker with olive oil, then add the cooked lamb, stock cube, rosemary, onion, garlic, salt, black pepper, and 3 cups of water. Blend to combine well.
3. Put the slow cooker lid on and cook on LOW for 8 hours.
4. Remove the cooked lamb stew from the slow cooker and serve warm.

TIP: To make this a complete meal, you can serve it with riced cauliflower and salmon salad.

PER SERVING
calories: 252 | total fat: 9.5g | carbs: 4.9g | protein: 34.9g

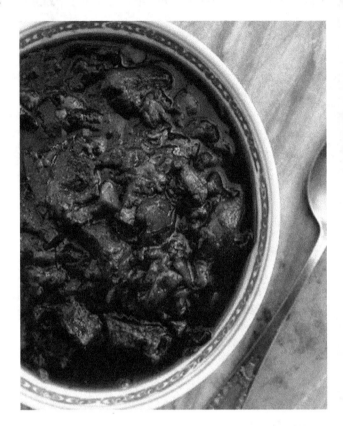

Ingredients:

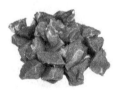

2 pounds (907 g) boneless lamb, cut into cubes

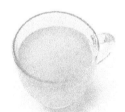

1 lamb stock cube

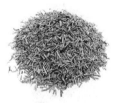

2 teaspoons dried rosemary

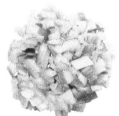

1 onion, roughly chopped

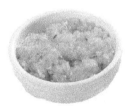

4 garlic cloves, finely chopped

FROM THE CUPBOARD:

Salt and freshly ground black pepper, to taste

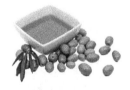

2 tablespoons olive oil, plus more for greasing the skillet

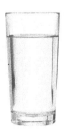

3 cups water

RICH ONION AND BEEF STEW

Macros: Fat 28% | Protein 68% | Carbs 4%

Prep time: 5 minutes | Cook time: 10 hours | Serves 6

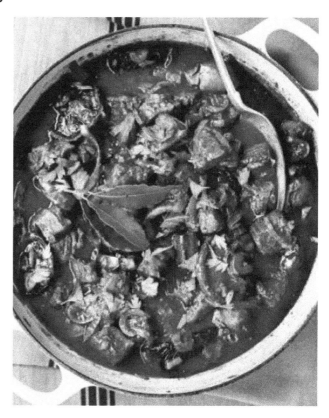

1. Grease the insert of the slow cooker with 2 tablespoons of olive oil. Coat a nonstick skillet with the remaining olive oil.
2. Heat the oil in the skillet over medium-high heat, then put the beef in the skillet and sear for 2 minutes or until medium-rare. Shake the skillet constantly to sear the beef cubes evenly.
3. Arrange the cooked beef in the slow cooker, then add the stock cube, mixed herbs, garlic, onions, salt, black pepper, and water. Stir to mix well.
4. Put the slow cooker lid on and cook on LOW for 10 hours.
5. Spoon the stew in a large bowl and serve warm.

TIP: To make this a complete meal, you can serve it with roasted broccoli or asparagus as the side dish.

PER SERVING
calories: 199 | total fat: 6.3g | carbs: 1.9g | protein: 33.8g

Ingredients:

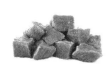

2 pounds (907 g) boneless stewing beef, cut into cubes

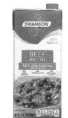

1 beef stock cube

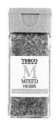

1 teaspoon dried mixed herbs (such as Italian seasoning)

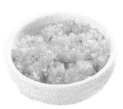

5 garlic cloves, crushed

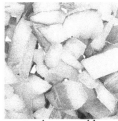

2 onions, roughly chopped

FROM THE CUPBOARD:

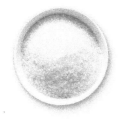

Salt and freshly ground black pepper, to taste

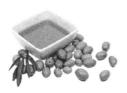

3 tablespoons olive oil, divided

SPECIAL EQUIPMENT:

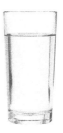

3 cups water

PORK STEW

Macros: Fat 44% | Protein 47% | Carbs 9%

Prep time: 5 minutes | Cook time: 8 hours | Serves 6

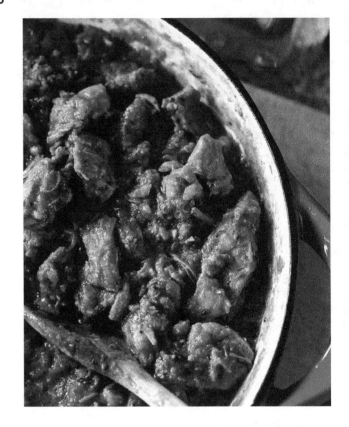

1. Grease the insert of the slow cooker with olive oil.
2. Mix the pork, chicken stock, onion, dried mixed spices, garlic, salt, and black pepper in the slow cooker.
3. Put the slow cooker lid on and cook on LOW for 8 hours.
4. Spoon the stew in a large bowl and serve warm.

TIP: To make this a complete meal, you can serve it with spinach salad or tomato and herb salad as the side dish.

PER SERVING
calories: 381 | total fat: 18.3g | carbs: 9.2g | protein: 42.3g

Ingredients:

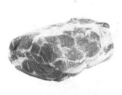

2 pounds (907 g) pork loin, cut into cubes

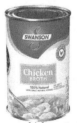

3 cups chicken stock

1 onion, finely chopped

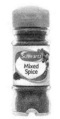

1 teaspoon dried mixed spices (homemade or store-bought)

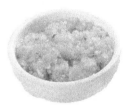

4 garlic cloves, crushed

FROM THE CUPBOARD:

Salt and freshly ground black pepper, to taste

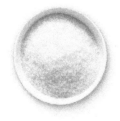

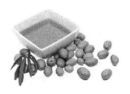

2 tablespoons olive oil

CAULIFLOWER AND CLAM CHOWDER

Macros: Fat 62% | Protein 27% | Carbs 11%

Prep time: 10 minutes | Cook time: 10 minutes | Serves 6

1. Divide the clams and clam juice into two bowls. Thin the clam juice with water to make 2 cups of juice.
2. Put the onion and butter in an instant pot and press the Sauté bottom, then sauté for 2 minutes or until the onion is translucent.
3. Add the clam juice and cauliflower into the instant pot. Put the lid on and press the Manual button, and set the temperature to 375°F (190°C), then cook for 5 minutes.
4. Quick Release the pressure, then open the lid and mix in the heavy cream and clams.
5. Press the Sauté bottom and cook for 3 minutes or until the clams are opaque and firm, then sprinkle with thyme, salt, and black pepper. Stir to mix well.
6. Spoon the chowder in a large bowl and serve warm.

TIP: To make this a complete meal, you can serve it with roasted bacon-wrapped chicken breasts.

PER SERVING
calories: 252 | total fat: 17.3g | total carbs: 8.9g | fiber: 2.1g | net carbs: 6.8g | protein: 17.1g

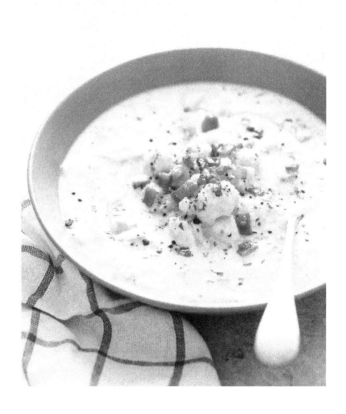

Ingredients:

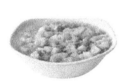

3 (6.5-ounce / 184-g) cans chopped clams

1 small yellow onion

4 cups chopped cauliflower

1½ cups heavy whipping cream

½ teaspoon dried thyme

FROM THE CUPBOARD:

Salt and freshly ground black pepper, to taste

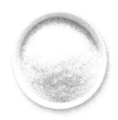

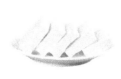

3 tablespoons butter

CHICKEN AND KALE SOUP

Macros: Fat 41% | Protein 45% | Carbs 14%

Prep time: 5 minutes | Cook time: 4 hours | Serves 4

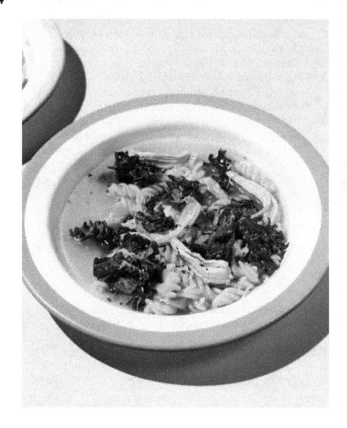

1. Grease the insert of the slow cooker with olive oil.
2. Mix the chicken breast, stock, kale, ginger, garlic, ginger, salt, and black pepper in the slow cooker.
3. Put the slow cooker lid on and cook on HIGH for 4 hours.
4. Spoon the stew in a large bowl and serve warm.

TIP: To make this a complete meal, you can serve it with roasted bacon-wrapped chicken breasts.

PER SERVING
calories: 168 | total fat: 7.6g | total carbs: 8.3g | fiber: 2.1g | net carbs: 6.2g | protein: 18.7g

Ingredients:

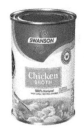

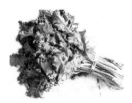

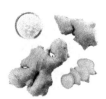

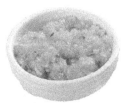

1 large chicken breast, cut into small strips	6 cups chicken stock	1 (7-ounce / 198-g) bunch kale, trimmed and chopped	3 tablespoons fresh ginger, grated	6 garlic cloves, finely chopped

FROM THE CUPBOARD:

Salt and freshly ground black pepper, to taste

2 tablespoons olive oil

CREAMY CELERY AND CHICKEN BROTH

Macros: Fat 65% | Protein 26% | Carbs 9%

Prep time: 5 minutes | Cook time: 20 minutes | Serves 4

1. Put the butter in a saucepan, and melt over medium heat.
2. Add and sauté the celery and onion for 3 minutes or until the onion is translucent.
3. Add the chicken, salt, black pepper, and water, and simmer for 15 minutes. Keep stirring during the simmering.
4. Stir in the coconut cream. Pour the soup in a large bowl and serve warm.

TIP: To make this a complete meal, you can serve it with riced cauliflower or zoodles.

PER SERVING
calories: 398 | total fat: 24.4g | net carbs: 5.9g | protein: 29.3g

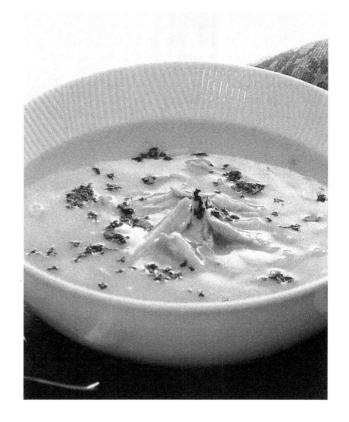

Ingredients:

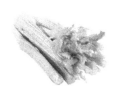

¼ cup celery, chopped

1 onion, chopped

2 chicken breasts, chopped

½ cup coconut cream

FROM THE CUPBOARD:

Salt and freshly ground black pepper, to taste

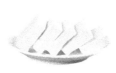

3 tablespoons butter

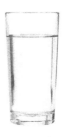

4 cups water

BUFFALO SAUCE AND TURKEY SOUP

Macros: Fat 65% | Protein 26% | Carbs 9%

Prep time: 5 minutes | Cook time: 10 minutes | Serves 4

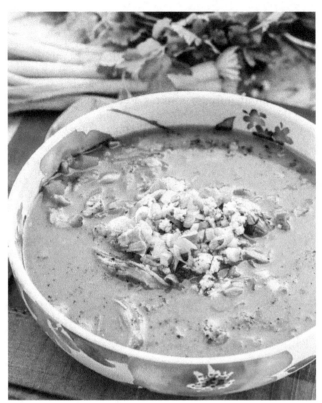

1. Put the buffalo sauce, cream cheese, and melted butter in a blender, and process until smooth.
2. Pour the buffalo sauce mixture in a saucepan, and add the chicken broth. Heat the soup over high heat until hot and almost boil but not boil. Keep stirring during the heating.
3. Add the shredded turkey, and sprinkle with salt and black pepper. Cook for 5 minutes or until smooth. Stir constantly.
4. Ladle the soup into a large bowl and top with chopped cilantro before serving.

TIP: To make this a complete meal, you can serve it with chicken and veggie skewers and a green salad.

PER SERVING
calories: 409 | total fat: 29.7g | net carbs: 9.2g | protein: 26.4g

Ingredients:

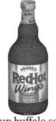

⅓ cup buffalo sauce

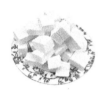

4 ounces (113 g) cream cheese

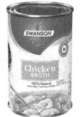

4 cups chicken broth

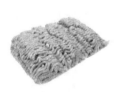

2 cups turkey, cooked, shredded

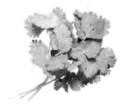

4 tablespoons cilantro, chopped

FROM THE CUPBOARD:

Salt and freshly ground black pepper, to taste

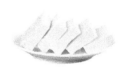

3 tablespoons butter, melted

SPECIAL EQUIPMENT:

MUSHROOM AND THYME SOUP

Macros: Fat 80% | Protein 9% | Carbs 11%

Prep time: 5 minutes | Cook time: 20 minutes | Serves 4

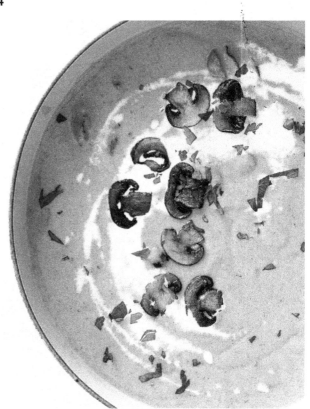

1. Put the butter in a saucepan and melt over medium heat.
2. Add the minced garlic and cook for 1 minutes or until fragrant.
3. Add the chopped mushrooms, and sprinkle with salt and black pepper. Stir to combine and cook for 10 minutes or until the mushrooms are tender.
4. Add the vegetable broth and bring the soup to a boil. Stir constantly. Lower the heat and simmer the soup for 10 minutes or until lightly thickened.
5. Pour the soup in a blender, and process until smooth, then fold in the crème fraiche.
6. Transfer the soup in a large bowl and top with thyme leaves before serving.

TIP: To make this a complete meal, you can serve it with beef stick and a green salad.

PER SERVING
calories: 282 | total fat: 25.1g | net carbs: 6.3g | protein: 7.8g

Ingredients:

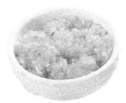

2 garlic cloves, minced

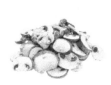

12 ounces (340 g) wild mushrooms, chopped

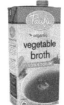

4 cups vegetable broth

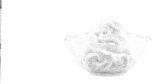

5 ounces (142 g) crème fraiche

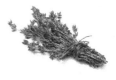

2 teaspoons thyme leaves

FROM THE CUPBOARD:

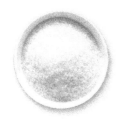

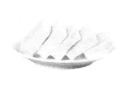

Salt and freshly ground black pepper, to taste   ¼ cup butter

SPECIAL EQUIPMENT:

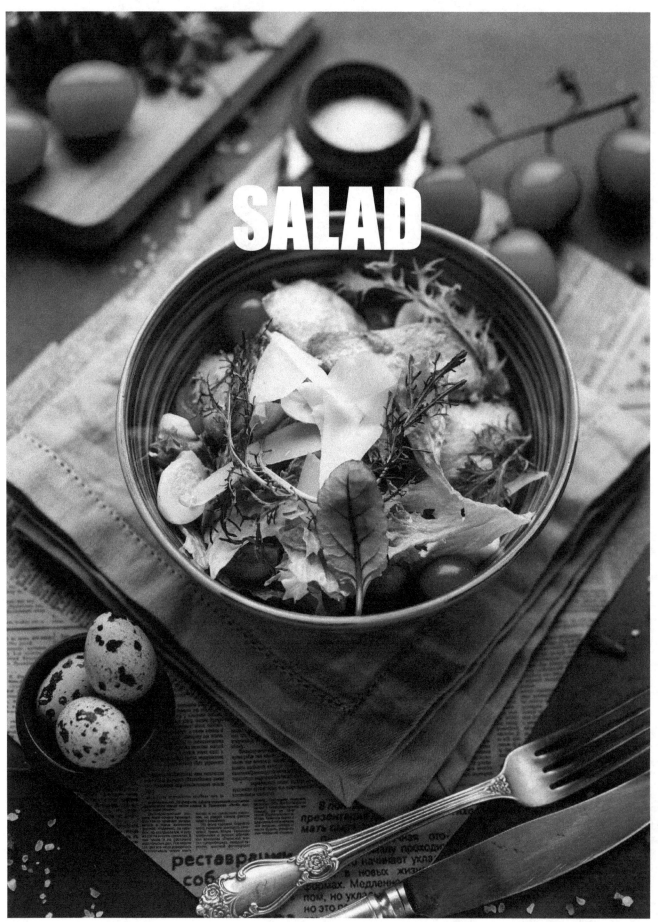

SALAD

CHEESE SALAD WITH BUTTERY VINEGAR

Macros: Fat 80% | Protein 18% | Carbs 2%

Prep time: 5 minutes | Cook time: 15 minutes | Serves 2

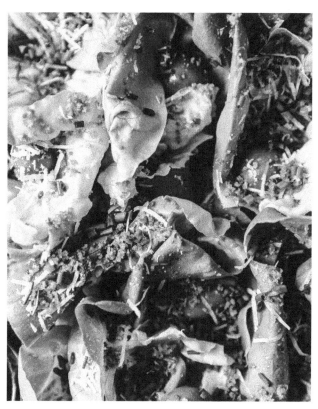

1. Preheat the oven to 400°F (205°C) and lightly grease a baking dish with the olive oil.
2. Place the goat cheese in the prepared baking dish. Arrange the baking dish in the preheated oven and bake for about 10 minutes until melted.
3. Meanwhile, in a frying pan over medium heat, toast the pumpkin seeds for about 5 to 7 minutes, or until the seeds turn a bit golden and start to pop, shaking the pan frequently to ensure even toasting.
4. Reduce the heat to medium-low, and add the butter. Cover, and simmer gently for a few minutes, or until you get a nice nutty scent. Pour in the balsamic vinegar and allow to boil for 2 to 3 minutes more until heated through. Remove from the heat to a bowl.
5. Remove the cheese from the oven. Divide the baby spinach between two plates, then top with the melted cheese. Serve it drizzled with the butter mixture.

TIP: The baby spinach can be replaced with lettuce for a distinct texture.

PER SERVING
calories: 821 | fat: 73.3g | protein: 37.2g | net carbs: 3.1g | fiber: 2g

Ingredients:

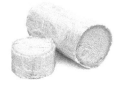

10 ounces (284 g) goat cheese, sliced

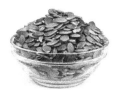

¼ cup pumpkin seeds

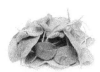

3 ounces (85 g) baby spinach

FROM THE CUPBOARD:

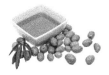

1 tablespoon olive oil, for greasing the baking dish

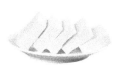

2 ounces (57 g) butter

1 tablespoon balsamic vinegar

FRIED ZUCCHINI SALAD

Macros: Fat 90% | Protein 4% | Carbs 6%

Prep time: 5 minutes | Cook time: 15 minutes | Serves 6

1. Put the zucchini pieces in a colander, then lightly sprinkle with the salt. Set aside for 5 to 10 minutes, pressing out the water.
2. In a skillet over medium heat, fry the zucchini in the olive oil for about 2 minutes until slightly softened. Remove from the heat and let cool for 5 minutes.
3. Once cooled, in a large bowl, combine the zucchini and remaining ingredients. Blend well. Serve immediately.

TIP: Store in an airtight container in the fridge for 2 to 3 days.

PER SERVING
calories: 320 | fat: 32.3g | protein: 3.2g | net carbs: 4.2g | fiber: 2g

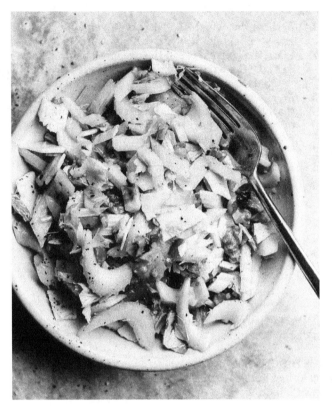

Ingredients:

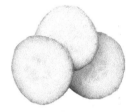

2 pounds (907 g) zucchini, peeled and seeds removed; cut into pieces, about ½ thick

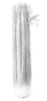

3 ounces (85 g) celery stalks, finely sliced

2 ounces (57 g) scallions, chopped

1 cup mayonnaise, keto-friendly

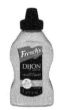

½ tablespoon Dijon mustard

FROM THE CUPBOARD:

Salt and pepper, to taste

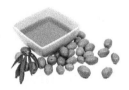

2 tablespoons olive oil

SIMPLE MOZZARELLA AND TOMATO SALAD

Macros: Fat 70% | Protein 25% | Carbs 5%

Prep time: 5 minutes | Cook time: 0 minutes | Serves 4

1. On a clean work surface, slice the Mozzarella balls and cherry tomatoes in half.
2. Transfer them to a bowl and fold in the pesto, then blend well. Season as needed with salt and pepper.
3. Serve at room temperature or refrigerate for 1 hour before serving.

TIP: To add more flavors to this meal, serve it topped with fresh basil or chives.

PER SERVING
calories: 225 | fat: 17.3g | protein: 14.2g | net carbs: 3.1g | fiber: 1g

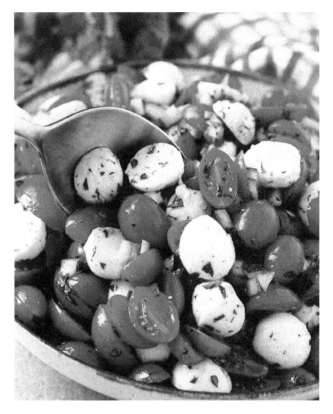

Ingredients:

8 ounces (227 g) Mozzarella, mini cheese balls

8 ounces (227 g) cherry tomatoes

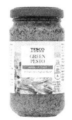

2 tablespoons green pesto

FROM THE CUPBOARD:

Salt and pepper, to taste

MANCHEGO AND PROSCIUTTO SALAD

Macros: Fat 90% | Protein 7% | Carbs 3%

Prep time: 5 minutes | Cook time: 10 minutes | Serves 2

1. Preheat the grill to low heat and lightly grease the grill grates with the olive oil.
2. Toss the lettuce with ½ cup olive oil in a bowl until coated well. Transfer the lettuce (face down) to the preheated grill.
3. Grill for about 2 minutes until the leaves are beginning to wilt. Flip the lettuce over and grill for 1 minute more.
4. Remove from the heat and allow to cool for 5 minutes.
5. On a flat work surface, slice the lettuce halves into smaller pieces.
6. Transfer the lettuce pieces to a bowl. Add the remaining olive oil, lemon juice, salt, and pepper. Toss well to incorporate.
7. Sprinkle the prosciutto pieces and shredded cheese on top, and serve.

TIP: For a unique twist, you can add a handful of toasted walnuts or almonds.

PER SERVING
calories: 1280.3 | fat: 128.3g | protein: 24.2g | net carbs: 7.2g | fiber: 8g

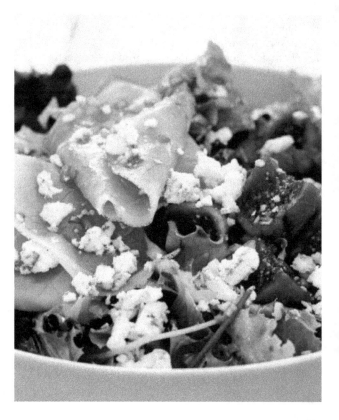

Ingredients:

3 ounces (85 g) manchego cheese, shredded

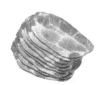

3 ounces (85 g) prosciutto, cut into bite-sized pieces

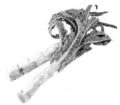

1 large head Romaine lettuce, cut in half

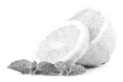

½ lemon, juiced

FROM THE CUPBOARD:

1 cup olive oil, plus more for greasing the grill grates

1 pinch salt

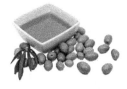

1 pinch ground black pepper

BROCCOLI AND MAYO SALAD WITH DILL

Macros: Fat 91% | Protein 4% | Carbs 5%

Prep time: 5 minutes | Cook time: 5 minutes | Serves 4

1. Put the broccoli florets in a pot of boiling salted water. Allow to boil for 3 to 4 minutes until lightly softened.
2. Remove from the heat. Drain the water and allow to cool.
3. In a large bowl, add the broccoli florets, mayo, and dill. Stir thoroughly until well combined.
4. Season as needed with salt and pepper, then serve.

TIP: The broccoli salad perfectly goes well with grilled chicken wings.

PER SERVING
calories: 417 | fat: 42.3g | protein: 4.1g | net carbs: 5.1g | fiber: 42g

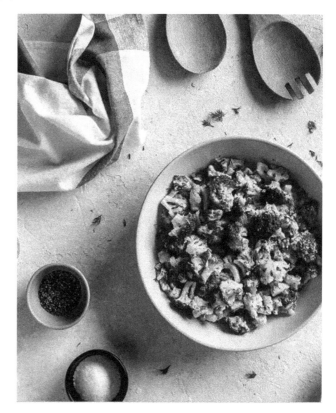

Ingredients:

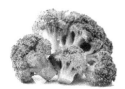

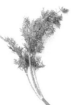

1 pound (454 g) broccoli, cut into small florets

1 cup mayonnaise, keto-friendly

¾ cup fresh dill

FROM THE CUPBOARD:

Salt and ground black pepper, to taste

KETO GREEN BEANS SALAD WITH AVOCADO

Macros: Fat 86% | Protein 6% | Carbs 8%

Prep time: 10 minutes | Cook time: 10 minutes | Serves 4

1. In a frying pan over medium-high heat, heat the olive oil.
2. Add the green beans and fry for 4 minutes, stirring frequently, or until the beans are bright green. Reduce the heat, and add the scallions. Season with salt and pepper, then transfer to a large bowl. Set aside.
3. In another bowl, using a fork to mash the avocados coarsely.
4. Put the mashed avocados and chopped onions into the bowl of green beans. Stir well.
5. Serve topped with the fresh cilantro.

TIP: You can also use the frozen green beans, making sure to thaw at room temperature before cooking.

PER SERVING
calories: 265 | fat: 25.3g | protein: 4.2g | net carbs: 5.2g | fiber: 9g

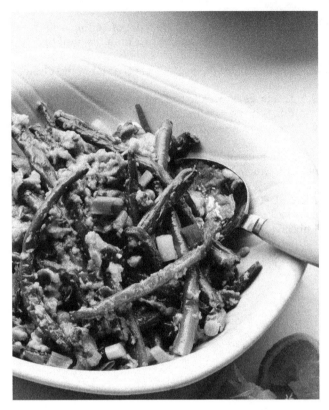

Ingredients:

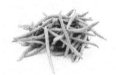

2/3 pound (299 g)fresh green beans, trimmed

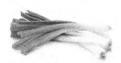

5 scallions

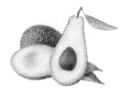

2 ripe avocados, peeled and pit removed

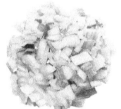

1 onion, chopped finely

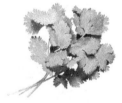

Handful of fresh cilantro, chopped finely

FROM THE CUPBOARD:

¼ teaspoon ground black pepper

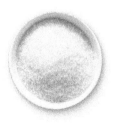

½ teaspoon sea salt

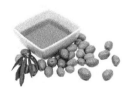

3 tablespoons olive oil

CREAMED SHRIMP SALAD

Macros: Fat 87% | Protein 11% | Carbs 2%

Prep time: 5 minutes | Cook time: 0 minutes | Serves 4

1. In a bowl, stir together the crème fraîche and mayo until smooth.
2. Add the chopped shrimp, fish roe, and lemon juice, salt and pepper. Whisk to combine.
3. Serve at room temperature or refrigerate for 1 hour before serving.

TIP: To add more flavors to this meal, top the salad with some lemon zest and Dijon mustard.

PER SERVING
calories: 500 | fat: 48.3g | protein: 14.2g | net carbs: 2.1g | fiber: 0g

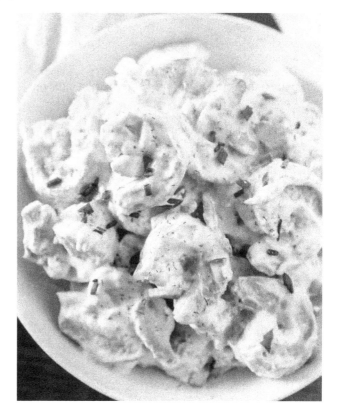

Ingredients:

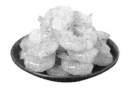

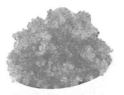

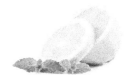

10 ounces (284 g) cooked shrimp, peeled and chopped roughly

¼ cup crème fraîche or sour cream

1 cup mayonnaise, keto-friendly

2 ounces (57 g) fish roe

2 teaspoons lemon juice

FROM THE CUPBOARD:

SPECIAL EQUIPMENT:

Salt and pepper, to taste

EASY ARUGULA SALAD

Macros: Fat 77% | Protein 16% | Carbs 7%

Prep time: 10 minutes | Cook time: 0 minutes | Serves 2

1. Add ½ tablespoon olive oil and arugula in a large bowl. Toss well. Sprinkle the salt and pepper to season.
2. Divide the seasoned arugula between two serving plates, then spread the sliced Mozzarella balls on top.
3. Top with the avocado, followed by the tomato slices. Pour the remaining olive oil over the arugula. Season with salt and pepper, if needed.
4. Serve sprinkled with the basil leaves.

TIP: The olive oil can be replaced with a vinaigrette dressing for a unique twist.

PER SERVING
calories: 318 | fat: 27.3g | protein: 13.1g | net carbs: 5.1g | fiber: 6g

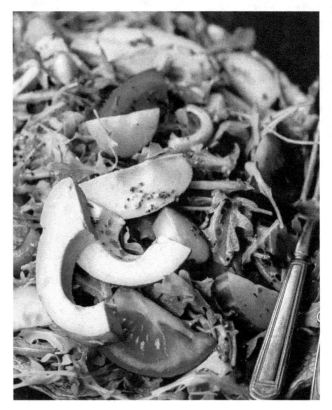

Ingredients:

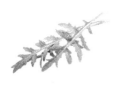

2 cups arugula

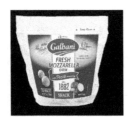

4 fresh Mozzarella balls, sliced

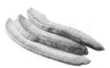

1 avocado, sliced

1 Roma tomato, sliced

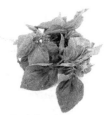

4 fresh basil leaves, cut into ribbons

FROM THE CUPBOARD:

SPECIAL EQUIPMENT:

Salt and freshly ground black pepper, to taste

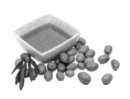

1 tablespoon olive oil, divided

SHRIMP AVOCADO WITH CELERY SALAD

Macros: Fat 64% | Protein 34% | Carbs 2%

Prep time: 5 minutes | Cook time: 2 minutes | Serves 2

1. Heat the olive oil in a large skillet over medium heat until sizzling.
2. Stir in the shrimp and fry for about 1 to 2 minutes until pink. Sprinkle the salt and pepper to taste.
3. Remove from the heat to a large bowl and cool for 5 minutes. Cover the bowl with plastic wrap, then place in the refrigerator for 10 minutes.
4. Stir together the celery, avocado, and mayo in a medium bowl until well combined. Sprinkle in the lime juice, salt and pepper. Mix well.
5. Remove the shrimp from the refrigerator to the medium bowl. Toss well to incorporate.
6. Cover the bowl with plastic wrap and refrigerate for about 30 minutes, then serve.

TIP: The salad perfectly goes well with the butter lettuce cups or romaine leaves.

PER SERVING
calories: 586 | fat: 41.3g | protein: 50.3g | net carbs: 3.3g | fiber: 5g

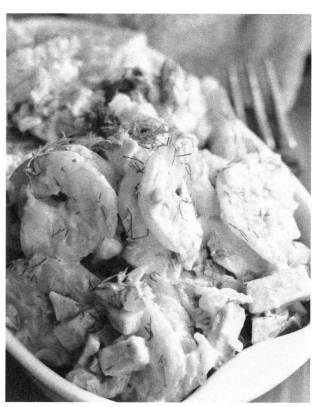

Ingredients:

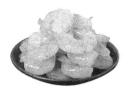

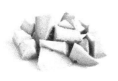

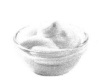

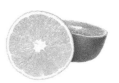

1 pound cooked shrimp (454 g), peeled and deveined, with tail off	1 avocado, cubed	1 celery stalk, chopped	¼ cup mayonnaise, keto-friendly	1 teaspoon freshly squeezed lime juice

FROM THE CUPBOARD:

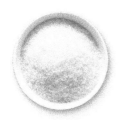

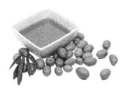

Salt and freshly ground black pepper, to taste

1 tablespoon olive oil, divided

ASPARAGUS WITH HARD-BOILED EGGS SALAD

Macros: Fat 82% | Protein 13% | Carbs 5%

Prep time: 20 minutes | Cook time: minutes | Serves 4

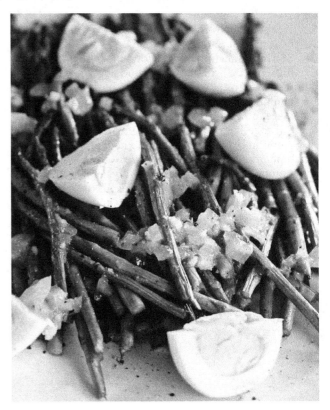

1. Make the dressing: Combine the vinegar, olive oil, and garlic in a small bowl. Add the salt and pepper, mix well. Set aside.
2. Using a vegetable peeler, shave the asparagus spears into thin ribbons, then place them in a bowl.
3. Make the salad: Add the pecans, eggs, and dressing into the bowl of asparagus. Toss thoroughly until combined well.
4. Evenly divide the salad among four serving plates, then serve.

TIP: This salad can be prepared ahead, but don't add the pecans or eggs until just before serving.

PER SERVING
calories: 255 | fat: 23.3g | protein: 8.2g | net carbs: 3.3g | fiber: 2g | sodium: 73mg

Ingredients:

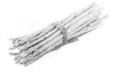

½ pound (227 g) asparagus stalks (about 20 medium), woody ends snapped off

4 hard-boiled eggs, peeled and chopped

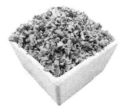

¼ cup pecans, chopped

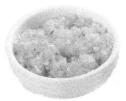

½ teaspoon garlic, minced

FROM THE CUPBOARD:

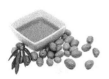

¼ cup olive oil

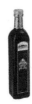

1½ tablespoons balsamic vinegar

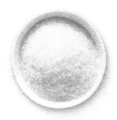

Sea salt, to taste

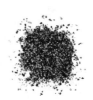

Freshly ground black pepper, to taste

CUCUMBER YOGURT RAITA SALAD WITH GRILLED TUNA

Macros: Fat 39% | Protein 52% | Carbs 9%

Prep time: 10 minutes | Cook time: 5 minutes | Serves 4

1. Put the cucumber slices in a bowl, and sprinkle with salt and pepper, then let stand to infuse for a few minutes.
2. Make the raita salad: Pat dry the seasoned cucumber with paper towels and put in a separate bowl. Add the mint, cumin, and yogurt to the bowl. Toss to combine well. Set aside until ready to serve.
3. Preheat the grill to high heat.
4. Arrange the tuna steaks on the preheated grill, and sprinkle with salt and pepper on both sides, then rub with olive oil on both sides.
5. Grill for 4 minutes or until it has been lightly cooked and has a pink in the center. Flip the tuna steaks halfway through the cooking time.
6. Transfer the fried tuna onto a platter and serve with raita salad.

TIP: To make this a complete meal, you can serve it with chicken and mushroom casserole. They also taste great paired with beef stew.

PER SERVING
calories: 379 | fat: 16.2g | fiber: 1.1g | net carbs: 7.8g | protein: 47.8g

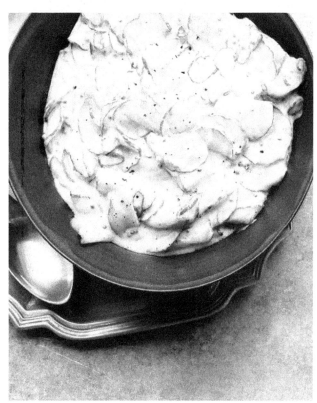

Ingredients:

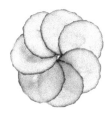

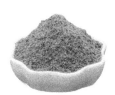

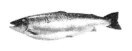

1½ pounds (680 g) cucumber, deseeded and cut into ½-inch (1.3-cm) slices	½ teaspoon ground cumin	2 tablespoons fresh mint	1¼ cups plain Greek yogurt	1½ pounds (680 g) fresh tuna, cut into 1-inch (2.5-cm) steaks

FROM THE CUPBOARD:

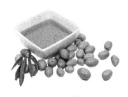

Salt and pepper, to taste   1 tablespoon olive oil

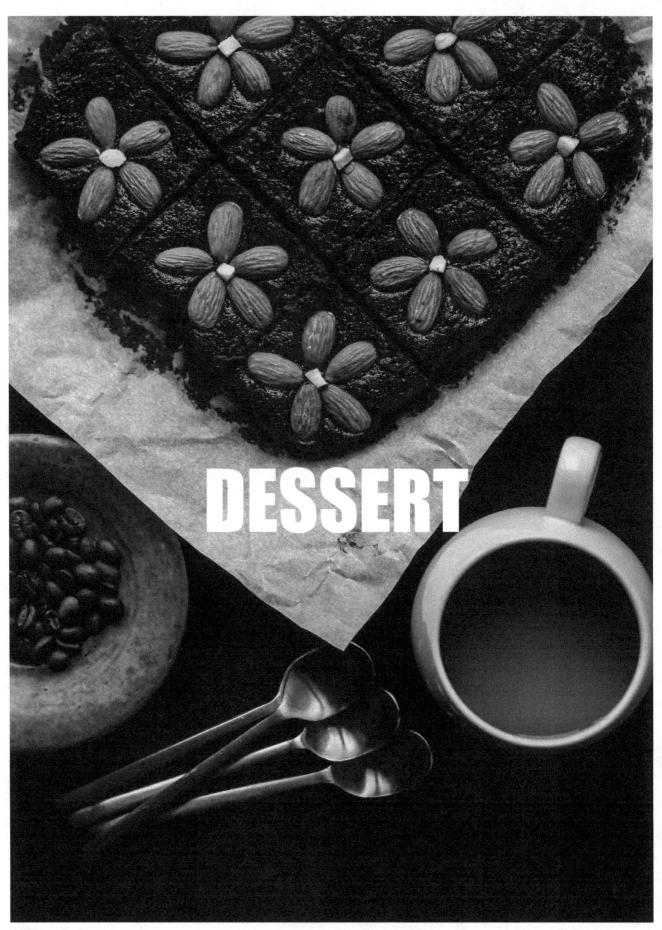

DESSERT

CHOCOLATE NUT BARS

Macros: Fat 88% | Protein 8% | Carbs 4%

Prep time: 60 minutes | Cook time: 0 minutes | Serves 16 bars

1. Line a baking pan with parchment paper.
2. Add all the ingredients to a food processor. Process until the mixture is coarse.
3. Pour the mixture evenly into the baking pan, then place the baking pan in the freezer to freeze for 45 minutes or until firm.
4. Remove the nut chunk from the freezer and cut into 16 bars to serve.

TIP: Store the bars in an airtight container in the fridge for up to 6 days, or in the freezer for up to 90 days.

PER SERVING
calories: 186 | total fat: 18.1g | fiber: 2.5g | net carbs: 1.7g | sugars: 0.7g | protein: 3.5g

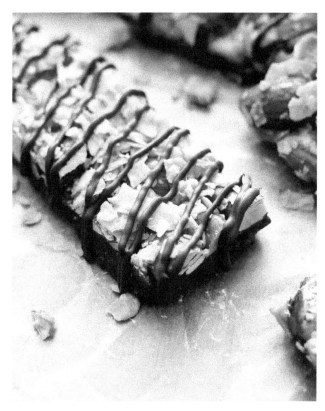

Ingredients:

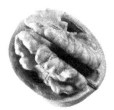

¼ cup walnuts

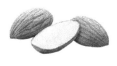

¼ cup almonds

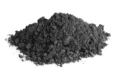

¼ cup cocoa powder

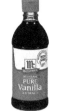

1 tablespoon pure vanilla extract

2 cups hazelnuts

FROM THE CUPBOARD:

1 teaspoon stevia powder

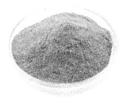

½ cup coconut oil

LEMONY BLUEBERRY CHOCOLATE CUPS

Macros: Fat 95% | Protein 2% | Carbs 3%

Prep time: 60 minutes | Cook time: 0 minutes | Serves 12 muffins

1. Add the coconut oil, and cocoa butter to a saucepan. Heat over medium-low heat. Keep stirring during the heating until combine well. Mix in the cocoa powder.
2. Turn the heat off, allow to cool for 10 minutes, then mix in the remaining ingredients.
3. Line a baking pan with 12 muffin paper cups.
4. Divide and spoon 1 tablespoon of the mixture into each muffin cups.
5. Place the baking pan into the fridge to chill for 45 minutes or until firm.
6. Remove the muffins from the fridge and serve chill.

TIP: Store the cups in an airtight container in the fridge for up to 6 days, or in the freezer for up to 90 days.

PER SERVING
calories: 179 | total fat: 18.9g | fiber: 1.2g | net carbs: 1.6g | sugars: 0.5g | protein: 0.7g

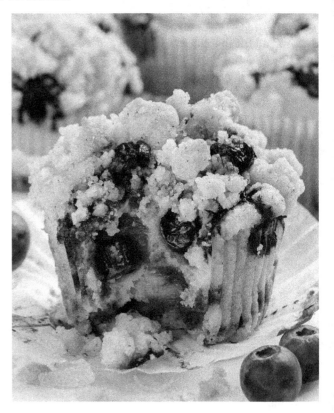

Ingredients:

½ cup cocoa butter

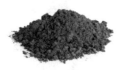

¼ cup cocoa powder

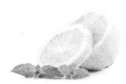

¼ cup fresh lemon juice

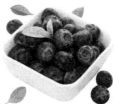

24 blueberries

2 tablespoons lemon zest

FROM THE CUPBOARD:

½ cup coconut oil

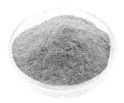

½ teaspoon stevia powder

MINT AND CHOCOLATE CUPS

Macros: Fat 89% | Protein 6% | Carbs 5%

Prep time: 60 minutes | Cook time: 0 minutes | Serves 16 cups

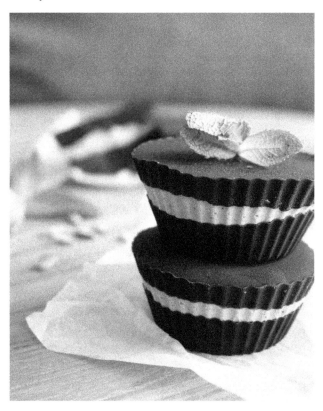

1. Add the almond butter, coconut oil, and cocoa butter to a saucepan. Heat over medium-low heat. Keep stirring during the heating until combine well. Mix in the cocoa powder.
2. Turn the heat off, allow to cool for 10 minutes, then mix in the remaining ingredients.
3. Line a baking pan with 16 muffin paper cups.
4. Divide and spoon 1 tablespoon of the mixture into each cups.
5. Place the baking pan into the fridge to chill for 45 minutes or until firm.
6. Remove the cups from the fridge and serve chill.

TIP: Store the cups in an airtight container in the fridge for up to 6 days, or in the freezer for up to 90 days.

PER SERVING
calories: 153 | total fat: 15.2g | fiber: 1.6g | net carbs: 1.2g | sugars: 0.3g | protein: 2.4g

Ingredients:

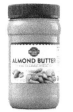

½ cup almond butter

½ cup cocoa butter

¼ cup unsweetened cocoa powder

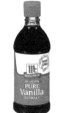

1 tablespoon vanilla extract

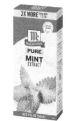

1 teaspoon mint extract

FROM THE CUPBOARD:

¼ cup coconut oil

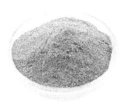

1 teaspoon stevia powder

CHOCOLATE FAT BOMBS

Macros: Fat 92% | Protein 4% | Carbs 4%

Prep time: 40 minutes | Cook time: 0 minutes | Serves 12 fat bombs

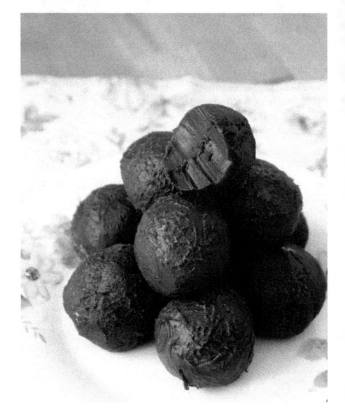

1. Line the parchment paper in a square cake tin.
2. Combine all the ingredients in a bowl, then pour the mixture into the cake tin.
3. Place the tin in the freezer to freeze for 30 minutes or until firm.
4. Remove the tin from the freezer and cut into 12 squares to serve.

TIP: You can store these chocolate bombs in an airtight container in the fridge for up to a week.

PER SERVING
calories: 117 | total fat: 11.9g | fiber: 1.6g | net carbs: 1.1g | sugars: 0.6g | protein: 1.3g

Ingredients:

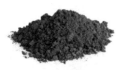

¼ cup unsweetened cocoa powder

½ cup coconut butter, melted

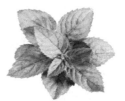

Fresh mint leaves, chopped

FROM THE CUPBOARD:

¼ cup coconut oil, melted

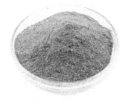

½ teaspoon stevia powder

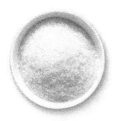

Salt, to taste

MATCHA CUPS

Macros: Fat 96% | Protein 2% | Carbs 2%

Prep time: 40 minutes | Cook time: 0 minutes | Serves 6

1. Line a 6-cup muffin tin with six cupcake papers.
2. Melt the coconut oil in a saucepan over low heat, then tile the saucepan so the coconut oil coat the bottom evenly.
3. Transfer the coconut oil to a large bowl, then mix in the remaining ingredients.
4. Pour the mixture in the six cups of the muffin tin, then place the tin in the freezer to freeze for 30 minutes before serving chill.

TIP: You can store the cups in an airtight container in the fridge for up to 5 days.

PER SERVING
calories: 379 | total fat: 40.6g | fiber: 0.7g | net carbs: 1.7g | sugars: 0.2g | protein: 1.4g

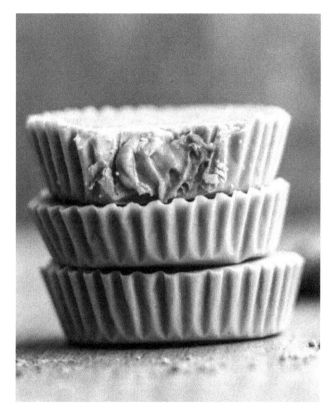

Ingredients:

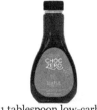

1 tablespoon low-carb maple syrup

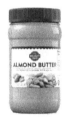

2 tablespoons almond butter

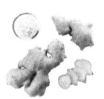

2-inch piece of ginger, finely grated

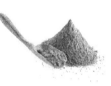

4 tablespoons matcha green tea powder

FROM THE CUPBOARD:

1 cup coconut oil

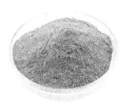

½ teaspoon stevia powder

Salt, to taste

SPECIAL EQUIPMENT:

A 6-cup muffin tin

CHEESECAKE WITH SOUR CREAM

Macros: Fat 83% | Protein 9% | Carbs 8%

Prep time: 15 minutes | Cook time: 20 minutes | Serves 6

1. Line a springform pan with parchment paper. Pour 2 cups of water into the pressure cooker. Place a trivet in the pressure cooker over the water.
2. Combine the cream cheese, lemon juice, ¼ cup of sour cream, ½ cup of sweetener, vanilla extract in a food processor. Process until the mixture is creamy and thick.
3. Break the eggs into the food processor and process for 20 to 30 seconds until the mixture is smooth.
4. Make the cheesecake: Pour the mixture in the springform pan, then cover with aluminum foil. Arrange the pan on the trivet in the pressure cooker.
5. Put the lid on and cook on HIGH for 20 minutes.
6. Meanwhile, combine the 2 tablespoons sweetener and remaining sour cream in a bowl.
7. Release the pressure in the pressure cooker, open the lid, and remove the aluminum foil. Top the cheesecake with the sweetener and sour cream mixture. Let the cheesecake sit for 10 minutes.
8. Place the cheesecake into the fridge to chill for at least 6 hours. Slice to serve.

TIP: The toppings of a cheesecake can be various, you can replace the mixture of sour cream and sweetener to shredded coconut, cocoa powder, or crushed walnuts. It mainly depends on your preference.

PER SERVING
calories: 208 | total fat: 19.2g | total carbs: 3.9g | fiber: 0g | net carbs: 3.9g | sugars: 1.9g | protein: 5.1g

Ingredients:

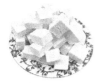
8 ounces (227 g) cream cheese

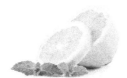
2 teaspoons freshly squeezed lemon juice

½ cup sour cream, divided

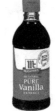
2 teaspoons vanilla extract

2 eggs

FROM THE CUPBOARD:

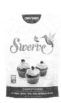
½ cup Swerve confectioners' style sweetener, plus 2 teaspoons

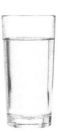
2 cups water

SPECIAL EQUIPMENT:

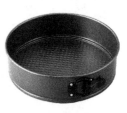
A springform pan

PANDAN AND COCONUT CUSTARD

Macros: Fat 80% | Protein 13% | Carbs 7%

Prep time: 10 minutes | Cook time: 30 minutes | Serves 4

1. Coat a heatproof bowl with melted butter.
2. Make the custard: Combine the beaten eggs, pandan extract, coconut milk, and stevia in a small bowl, then pour the mixture into the heatproof bowl.
3. Cover the bowl of mixture with aluminum foil. Pour 2 cups of water into the pressure cooker. Place a trivet in the pressure cooker over the water.
4. Arrange the bowl on the trivet, then put the lid on and cook on HIGH for 30 minutes or until the eggs are set and no longer jiggle.
5. Release the pressure, then open the lid and remove the bowl from the pressure cooker. Remove the aluminum foil and allow to cool for 10 minutes.
6. Transfer the bowl into the fridge and chill for 6 hours before serving.

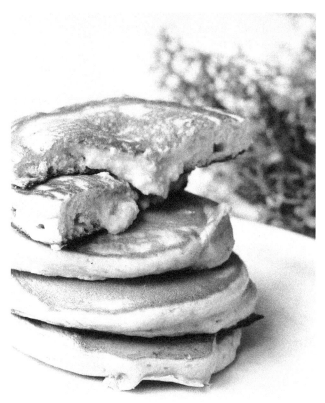

TIP: You can serve this pandan and coconut custard with chocolate puddings or berry smoothies.

PER SERVING
calories: 204 | total fat: 18.2g | total carbs: 3.9g | fiber: 1.0g | net carbs: 2.9g | sugars: 1.9g | protein: 5.9g

Ingredients:

3 eggs, beaten

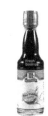

2 teaspoons pandan extract

1 cup unsweetened coconut milk

FROM THE CUPBOARD:

2 tablespoons melted butter

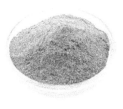

1 teaspoon stevia powder

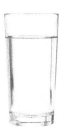

2 cups water

ZUCCHINI KHEER

Macros: Fat 80% | Protein 10% | Carbs 10%

Prep time: 5 minutes | Cook time: 10 minutes | Serves 4

1. Combine the heavy cream, zucchini, coconut milk, and xylitol in a pressure cooker.
2. Put the lid on and cook on HIGH for 10 minutes.
3. Release the pressure, then open the lid and fold in the cardamom.
4. Transfer them into a large bowl and serve warm.

TIP: To make this a complete meal, you can serve it with curry chicken and curry mushroom and broccoli.

PER SERVING
calories: 70 | total fat: 8.3g | total carbs: 3.5g | fiber: 0.1g | net carbs: 2.4g | sugars: 3.2g | protein: 2.5g

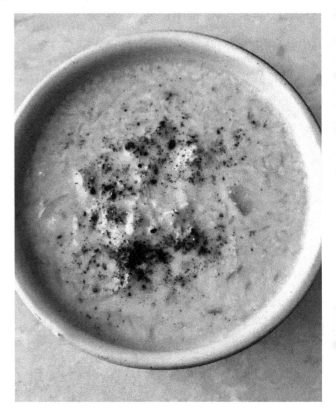

Ingredients:

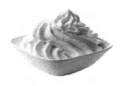

5 ounces (142 g) heavy whipping cream

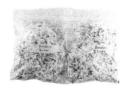

2 cups shredded zucchini

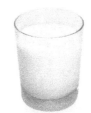

5 ounces (142 g) coconut milk

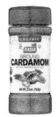

½ teaspoon ground cardamom

FROM THE CUPBOARD:

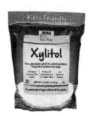

¼ cup xylitol

CAULIFLOWER, PEANUT, ALMOND, AND COCONUT SMOOTHIE

Macros: Fat 66% | Protein 20% | Carbs 14%

Prep time: 10 minutes | Cook time: 0 minutes | Serves 2

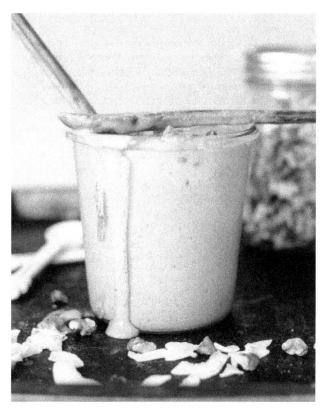

1. Put the cauliflower, almond milk, peanut butter, coconut milk, and protein powder in a blender, then process until well combined and creamy.
2. Add the ice cubes in the blender and process until smooth.
3. Divide the mixture into two glasses and serve chill.

TIP: Smoothie is a perfect drink to serve with all kinds of food, the texture and the chill of it can bring you a totally different palate enjoyment while enjoying with other dishes. You can try to make the smoothies with berries or some vegetables such as tomatoes.

PER SERVING
calories: 396 | total fat: 29.2g | total carbs: 12.9g | fiber: 7.1g | net carbs: 5.8g | protein: 19.6g

Ingredients:

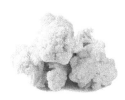

1 cup cooked cauliflower

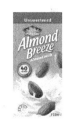

½ cup unsweetened almond milk

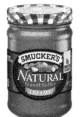

2 tablespoons natural peanut butter

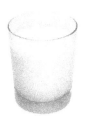

½ cup coconut milk

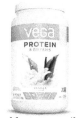

1 tablespoon vanilla protein powder

FROM THE CUPBOARD:

3 ice cubes

CHIA SEEDS AND BLACK BERRY PUDDING

Macros: Fat 78% | Protein 7% | Carbs 15%

Prep time: 10 minutes | Cook time: 0 minutes | Serves 2

1. Combine the vanilla extract, coconut milk, and stevia in a food processor.
2. Add the blackberries and pulse the food processor until smooth, then mix in the chia seeds.
3. Pour the mixture into two cups with lids, then arrange them in the refrigerator and chill for at least 8 hours.
4. Remove the cups from the refrigerator and serve the puddings chill.

TIP: Pudding can be used in various ways, for example, you can serving the pudding on top of trifles or smoothies to gift flavor.

PER SERVING
calories: 439 | total fat: 38.2g | total carbs: 22.8g | fiber: 15.3g | net carbs: 7.5g | protein: 7.8g

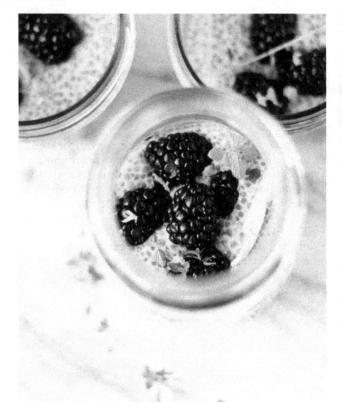

Ingredients:

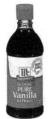

1 teaspoon vanilla extract

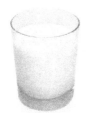

1 cup unsweetened full-fat coconut milk

½ cup blackberries (fresh or frozen)

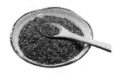

¼ cup chia seeds

FROM THE CUPBOARD:

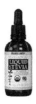

1 teaspoon liquid stevia

BLACKBERRY AND BLUEBERRY ICE POPS

Macros: Fat 93% | Protein 3% | Carbs 4%

Prep time: 5 minutes | Cook time: 0 minutes | Serves 2

1. Combine the vanilla extract, coconut cream, and sweetener in a blender.
2. Add the mixed berries to the blender. Process until the mixture is smooth.
3. Pour the mixture into the ice pop molds. Put them into the freezer for 2 hours, then serve chill.

TIP: You can increase the quantity of the ingredients to make more ice pops each time.

PER SERVING
calories: 167 | total fat: 17.2g | total carbs: 3.9g | fiber: 1.5g | net carbs: 2.3g | protein: 1.2g

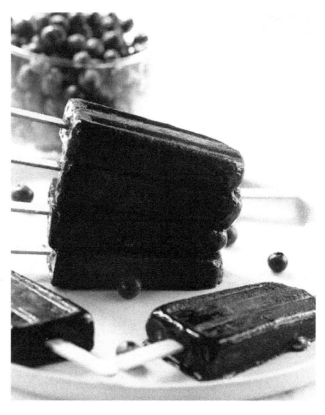

Ingredients:

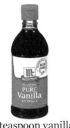

½ teaspoon vanilla extract

½ (13.5-ounce / 383-g) can coconut cream

¼ cup mixed blackberries and blueberries (fresh or frozen)

FROM THE CUPBOARD:

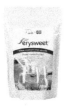

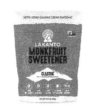

2 teaspoons monk fruit sweetener or erythritol

SPECIAL EQUIPMENT:

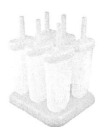

Ice pop molds

LEMONY STRAWBERRY ICE POPS

Macros: Fat 92% | Protein 3% | Carbs 5%

Prep time: 5 minutes | Cook time: 0 minutes | Serves 2

1. Combine the lime juice, coconut milk, and stevia in a blender.
2. Add the strawberries to the blender. Process until the mixture is smooth.
3. Pour the mixture into the ice pop molds. Put them into the freezer for 2 hours, then serve chill.

TIP: You can increase the quantity of the ingredients to make more ice pops each time.

PER SERVING
calories: 168 | total fat: 17.2g | total carbs: 4.9g | fiber: 1.2g | net carbs: 3.7g | protein: 1.1g

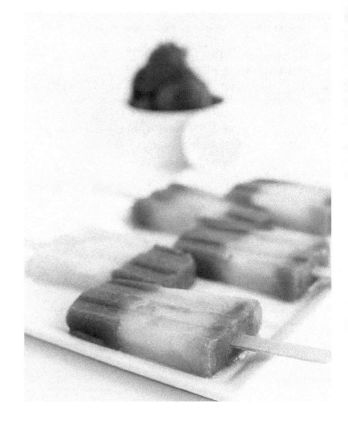

Ingredients:

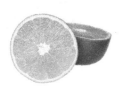

1 tablespoon freshly squeezed lime juice

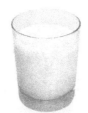

¾ cup unsweetened full-fat coconut milk

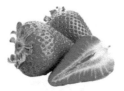

¼ cup hulled and sliced strawberries (fresh or frozen)

FROM THE CUPBOARD:

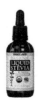

1 teaspoon liquid stevia

SPECIAL EQUIPMENT:

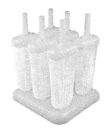

Ice pop molds

MEASUREMENT CONVERSION CHART

VOLUME EQUIVALENTS(DRY)

US STANDARD	METRIC (APPROXIMATE)
1/8 teaspoon	0.5 mL
1/4 teaspoon	1 mL
1/2 teaspoon	2 mL
3/4 teaspoon	4 mL
1 teaspoon	5 mL
1 tablespoon	15 mL
1/4 cup	59 mL
1/2 cup	118 mL
3/4 cup	177 mL
1 cup	235 mL
2 cups	475 mL
3 cups	700 mL
4 cups	1 L

VOLUME EQUIVALENTS(LIQUID)

US STANDARD	US STANDARD (OUNCES)	METRIC (APPROXIMATE)
2 tablespoons	1 fl.oz.	30 mL
1/4 cup	2 fl.oz.	60 mL
1/2 cup	4 fl.oz.	120 mL
1 cup	8 fl.oz.	240 mL
1 1/2 cup	12 fl.oz.	355 mL
2 cups or 1 pint	16 fl.oz.	475 mL
4 cups or 1 quart	32 fl.oz.	1 L
1 gallon	128 fl.oz.	4 L

WEIGHT EQUIVALENTS

US STANDARD	METRIC (APPROXIMATE)
1 ounce	28 g
2 ounces	57 g
5 ounces	142 g
10 ounces	284 g
15 ounces	425 g
16 ounces (1 pound)	455 g
1.5 pounds	680 g
2 pounds	907 g

TEMPERATURES EQUIVALENTS

FAHRENHEIT(F)	CELSIUS(C) (APPROXIMATE)
225 °F	107 °C
250 °F	120 °C
275 °F	135 °C
300 °F	150 °C
325 °F	160 °C
350 °F	180 °C
375 °F	190 °C
400 °F	205 °C
425 °F	220 °C
450 °F	235 °C
475 °F	245 °C
500 °F	260 °C

References

098photoshootings. (2017, Jan. 15). Couple cooking together. Pixabay. https://pixabay.com/photos/woman-kitchen-man-everyday-life-1979272/

Annekroiss. (2020, Mar. 3). Frozen berries. Pixabay. https://pixabay.com/photos/frozen-berries-blackberry-frost-4896919/

Congerdesign. (2014, Nov. 25). Kitchen equipment. Pixabay. https://pixabay.com/photos/pot-kitchen-cook-wooden-spoon-544071/

Congerdesign. (2016, Dec. 12). Knife block. Pixabay. https://pixabay.com/photos/knife-block-knife-kitchen-cook-1897410/

Couleur. (2016, Aug. 16). Olive oil bottle. Pixabay. https://pixabay.com/photos/olive-oil-oil-food-carafe-1596639/

Engin_Akyurt. (2020, Apr. 18). Bakery breads. Pixabay. https://pixabay.com/photos/bread-grain-carb-food-wheat-fresh-5054901/

Felix_w. (2018, Oct. 23). Steak in a cast iron pan. Pixabay. https://pixabay.com/photos/steak-pan-rosemary-food-meat-beef-3766548/

Frank, G. (2016, Sept. 14). Why fat in your diet is good for weight loss, glowing skin and more. Today. https://www.today.com/health/why-fat-your-diet-good-weight-loss-glowing-skin-t102800

Free-Photos. (2015, Nov. 10). Burger ingredients. Pixabay. https://pixabay.com/photos/hamburger-cheeseburger-ingredients-1030865/

Gadini. (2015, Aug. 2). Thermometer. Pixabay. https://pixabay.com/photos/thermometer-temperature-measurement-869392/

GamerChef6. (2016, Sept. 15). Grocery list. Pixabay. https://pixabay.com/photos/grocery-list-pen-paper-notepad-1670408/

JillWellington. (2015, June 1). Vegetable harvest. Pixabay. https://pixabay.com/photos/vegetables-garden-harvest-organic-790022/

LisaRedfern. (2015, Dec. 14). Pecans. Pixabay. https://pixabay.com/photos/pecan-toasted-nuts-candied-nuts-1090266/

MaineWoodsChick. (2019, June 5). Jarred goods. Pixabay. https://pixabay.com/photos/canned-canning-farm-stand-mason-jar-4251790/

Pexels. (2016, Nov. 19). Cutting board with ingredients. Pixabay. https://pixabay.com/photos/avocado-chopping-board-cooking-eggs-1838785/

Pexels. (2016, Nov. 20). Handful of beans. Pixabay. https://pixabay.com/photos/runner-beans-food-people-daytime-1835646/

Pinto, C. (n.d.). Leftovers. Unsplash. https://unsplash.com/photos/2lWGQ02DGL8

Ponce_photography. (2016, June 8). Strawberry yogurt. Pixabay. https://pixabay.com/photos/yogurt-fruit-vanilla-strawberries-1442034/

Silviarita. (2017, May 12). Fruit salad. Pixabay. https://pixabay.com/photos/fruit-fruits-fruit-salad-fresh-bio-2305192/

Stevepb. (2015, Oct. 5). Olive oil dressing. Pixabay. https://pixabay.com/photos/olive-oil-salad-dressing-cooking-968657/

Stevepb. (2015, Aug. 14). Spices and seasonings. Pixabay. https://pixabay.com/photos/spices-flavorings-seasoning-food-887348/

Dear Readers and Friends:

This is an invitation to step closer to us by voicing your opinion about our book. We are a group of dietitians and nutritionists who are so keen about diets, nutrition, and lifestyle that we have devoted our past 6 years researching, developing, testing, and writing recipes and cookbooks. This is the profession we take so much pride in, and we strive to write high-quality recipes and produce value-packed cookbooks. If you like our books, please do us a favor and leave an objective, honest and detailed review on our amazon page, the more specific, the better! It may take only a couple of minutes, but would mean the world to us. We will never stop devoting our careers and minds to producing more high-quality cookbooks to serve you better.

Additionally, You can get one book named keto diet mistakes for beginners as a free bonus from the link: https://mailchi.mp/0c3fd48025c3/keto-diet-cookbook, it would be appreciated if you like it.

CPSIA information can be obtained
at www.ICGtesting.com
Printed in the USA
BVHW011851170521
607567BV00003B/25